The Healthy Hundred

The Healthy Hundred

100 Ways to a Healthier, Happier and Longer Life

Dr PETER A. LARKINS

WILEY

First published in 2024 by John Wiley & Sons Australia, Ltd
Level 4, 600 Bourke St, Melbourne, Victoria 3000, Australia

Typeset in Baskerville URW 11pt/16pt

ISBN: 978-1-394-21608-6

 A catalogue record for this book is available from the National Library of Australia

Cover design and colour wheel graphic by Alex Ross Creative

Disclaimer

SKY9F15F25B-F6D6-421A-B6C2-2AC6C5546D3D_032024

For Thomas, Charlie and Jeremy, with love

Contents

Foreword by Eddie McGuire   *xiii*

About the author   *xix*

Acknowledgements   *xxi*

Introduction   *xxiii*

Part I: Taking a pulse check on aging and good health   **1**

1   Moving from aging to healthspan   3

2   Your health: Whose responsibility is it?   13

Part II: Monitoring your health   **21**

3   Key medical conditions to understand — and avoid   23

4   Health issues for men and women   49

5   Checking your health — the why, how and when   67

Part III: 100 ways to improve your healthspan   **77**

6   Exercise   79

    Exercise — the most important medicine you can take   *79*

    #1   Learn how exercise works to improve health   81

    #2   Use exercise as the ultimate health supplement   83

    #3   Work out if you need medical screening   84

    #4   Seek advice on planning your best exercise program   87

    #5   Know how to start an exercise program   88

#6 Understand what motivates you to improve your fitness 92

#7 Know your limits and keep exercise safe 94

#8 Find time for exercise 95

#9 Don't let excuses get in your way 97

#10 Start with small changes for big gains 99

#11 Take some time for recovery 100

#12 Prepare your workout clothes the night before 101

#13 Increase your walking speed 103

#14 Get those steps in 104

#15 Boost your mitochondria 105

#16 Increase your NAD 108

#17 Increase your lifespan — and healthspan — with exercise 109

7 Nutrition 113

Food – a critical component of healthy living 114

#18 Focus on your gut health 114

#19 Know the fuel your body needs 117

#20 Balance your food intake for body and brain 118

#21 Choose foods that are best for your brain and body 120

#22 Avoid processed foods 125

#23 Focus on good carbohydrates 126

#24 Build and repair with protein 127

#25 Know your good fats and bad fats 128

#26 Cut your sugar 130

#27 Eat some chocolate! 133

#28 Use salt sparingly 135

Good fluid intake and hydration 137

#29 Appreciate water — understand why you need it and how much 137

#30 Enhance performance with milk 140

#31 Boost your heart health with moderate
coffee consumption 143

#32 Enjoy a cup of tea 148

#33 Watch your alcohol consumption 150

Your diet and you 151

#34 Aim for a healthy, sustainable weight 152

#35 Take some tips from the Mediterranean diet 153

#36 Pursue your (nutrition) rainbow 157

#37 Benefit from fasting and timed eating 161

#38 Snack well 163

#39 Reduce your inflammation 164

#40 Consider supplements — maybe 166

#41 Understand food labelling 171

#42 Masticate more — and slowly 172

8 Habits 175

Look after yourself with everyday simple actions 175

#43 Make sure you get enough sleep 176

#44 Focus on your sleep hygiene 180

#45 Watch out for sleep deficit and sleep deprivation 181

#46 Monitor your sleep 182

#47 Avoid sleep disorders 182

#48 Dream sweetly 187

#49 Get your daily DOSE of happy hormones 190

#50 Breathe easy 196

#51 Quit smoking — right now! 198

#52 Protect your skin — health is more than skin deep 201

Use it, train it, nourish it – or lose it 203

#53 Get moving every day—incidental activity 204

#54 Stand up for yourself 205

#55 Take the stairs 207

#56 Adjust your parking habits 208

#57 Own a dog! 209

#58 Look after your joints—they keep you moving 212

#59 Get treated for osteoarthritis pain 216

#60 Set an exercise challenge 220

#61 Find your preferred cardio option 222

#62 Chill out with cold immersion 223

Working out where you are in life 225

#63 Understand why postcodes matter 226

#64 Live near a defibrillator 227

#65 Minimise jet lag 228

#66 Get a dose of sunshine—but stay sun smart 230

#67 Be beside the seaside—or any good view 232

#68 Keep up to date with your vaccinations 233

#69 Know your family history 235

9 Mindset 239

Focus on yourself – and nurture others 239

#70 Manage your stress 240

#71 Recognise and avoid burnout 247

#72 Build your willpower (and avoid the 'won't power') 249

#73 Don't be too hard on yourself 251

#74 Think like a child 252

#75 Practise gratefulness 254

#76 Be selfish—it's not always a bad choice! 255

#77   Never stop learning   257

#78   Set your goals   258

#79   Pay attention to the detail   260

#80   Avoid procrastination   262

#81   Learn the value of solitude   264

#82   Practise compassion   265

#83   Seek out mentors   266

#84   Scrutinise expert opinion   271

#85   Get a good financial planner   274

#86   Pick your battles   276

#87   Learn to adapt   278

#88   Know it's never too early to start — or too late   280

#89   Keep everything in moderation   283

10   Connection   285

The importance of family, friendship and community   285

#90   Get married!   286

#91   Enjoy a healthy sex life   288

#92   Instil healthy habits in your children   291

#93   Keep in mind that laughter really is medicinal   295

#94   Take advantage of the benefits of drinking wine   297

#95   Have a hobby   302

#96   Listen to whatever is music to your ears   304

#97   Plan a holiday   305

#98   Enjoy the perfect holiday with the seven Ss   307

#99   Have a workout buddy   314

#100 Never judge a book by its cover   315

Conclusion: What now?   319

Index   325

Foreword by Eddie McGuire

'Your job is to keep me alive!'

It would appear I wasn't the only one saying this to my long-time colleague and friend Dr Peter Larkins.

Broken bones, exhaustion, general maladies and the effects of going from 'bullet proof' to 'less bullet proof' over the years, Dr Larkins has seen and largely fixed all this and more. He is my go-to man in the media, personally and for friends and family.

When something goes wrong, 'Ring Dr Peter.'

Peter has a unique combination of skills and idiosyncrasies.

He possesses an athlete's ruthless dedication, a physician's clear thinking, a scientist's approach to problem solving, a natural raconteur's ear for a good story and he communicates with ease.

He also has that old-style 'missionary' approach to helping people and throwing himself at worthy causes.

I first spotted Peter in action in 1977 at, of all places, the Melbourne Cricket Ground, during what has become one of the most iconic sports events, the Centenary Test of Cricket.

Long before the likes of Robbie Williams provided pre-match entertainment at major sporting events, the organisers of the day had a local band on the back of a flatbed truck doing laps of the famous ground.

The other crowd occupier during the break in play for lunch was a mile race around the ground featuring the super athlete of the day, New Zealander, Olympic champion and world record holder, John Walker. Competing against the great man, the Australian 3000 metre steeplechase champion, a young doctor from Geelong: Peter Larkins.

The locals did well until the superstar of world athletics, Walker, took off for home, long hair flowing in his slipstream as he strode over the line in first place.

For a 12-year-old boy watching from the stands, that was some day.

That day Rod Marsh made 95 not out, debutant David Hookes hit the English captain Tony Greig for five boundaries in a row, and Australian batsman Rick McCosker, having been felled in the first innings by a bouncer that smashed into his face, returned to the crease with a broken jaw, his face covered in bandages, as the crowd sang 'Waltzing McCosker'.

Anyone who graced the field that day was a legend to me!

So, as the years went on, the name Dr Peter Larkins would pop-up and I'd remember him being part of that great day in the history of sport.

And pop-up it did. As the athlete who went on to win seven Australian Championships and represent his country at the Olympic Games, the World Championships and the Commonwealth Games, and then popping up more often as an expert physician.

And then, when I started in the media, Peter Larkins was one of the most respected names in sports medicine as AFL club doctor at Geelong and Adelaide (among his many sporting positions) and later as the president of the Sports Medicine Association of Australia.

In that role Peter became a constant source of information.

When the opportunity came to put together the Triple M Football broadcasting team, and later the groundbreaking AFL on Nine team, I had no hesitation in asking Dr Peter to be our medical expert.

Previously, the role of 'boundary rider' had gone to a colourful former footballer, but we decided that, as injuries were such a major part of the game, a 'real expert' was required. This person needed medical expertise, an understanding of top-line competitive sport, the ability to break a story, to be unflinching in his honesty and to understand the theatre of live sport.

Enter 'Dr Peter Larkins on the boundary.'

Peter Larkins changed the role forever.

Instead of waiting until 'next week' for medical updates, Peter's contacts and instant observation diagnosis changed the face of broadcasting.

It was not unusual for football clubs to ask him for his clinical diagnosis or to help 'pop back in' a dislocated shoulder or two while holding his microphone.

Peter turned what had been a ham-fisted, euphemism-laden part of broadcasting into pure journalism and changed the nature of covering sport from a medical point of view forever.

What is most pertinent to the writing of this book is his constant attendance at medical symposiums around the world, which has kept Peter at the forefront of world practices.

If there is one area of medical science that is always trying, often too hard, it is sports medicine.

Peter has been at the forefront of world sports medicine for over three decades. This, added to his burgeoning practice, has given him not only a theoretical leading position, but a hands-on daily connection to his patients.

In other words, he's seen it all and heard it all.

So when I say to Peter, 'Your job is to keep me alive!', I do so in the confidence that he's up to date on everything from the latest internet or celebrity fad, to new and improved, clinically-tested regimes, and has sorted through the brilliant from the bull!

I hope you enjoy this book as much as I have.

Some of what Peter writes is self-evident and well known, and for good reason: it works.

Sometimes the 'secret' is pretty straightforward: sleep, food and exercise...who would have thought? But Pete's other well-learned lessons of fun, drive and purpose in life sets a pretty compelling structure to getting to the big 100!

His media colleagues might call him Dr Smooth and Doc Hollywood because of his proficiency behind the microphone, but I always regard Dr Peter Larkins as Dr Sincerity. With Pete, you know he's always doing his best for you and usually when you need a friend, and an expert one at that.

Who knows, with a bit of luck and medical advancements, we might get to the 'Bi-Centenary of Test Cricket'!

Here's to a life well-lived.

Eddie McGuire

About the author

Dr Peter Larkins has been involved in the health and fitness industry his entire life.

From his beginnings as the inspiration for the popular Little Athletics movement in Australia to an international career as an Olympian, World Cup and Commonwealth Games athlete, he has always focused on healthy living practices and the pursuit of high performance — in sport and in all aspects of life.

During his 10-year international competitive career, he completed degrees in medicine and exercise physiology, before receiving travelling scholarships to pursue post graduate study overseas.

His sporting life fueled his interest in all aspects of human performance including the physiology of fitness, nutrition, sports injury management and the mental approaches to achieve at the highest level.

Peter established the first solo specialist sports physician practice in Australia and has served on numerous government and organisational advisory committees. He is past National President of Sports Medicine Australia — the peak advisory group on fitness, health and sport in Australia. He has been team physician for many sports including the Australian cricket team, triathlon, lacrosse and track and field teams. He also worked as a medical officer with the Geelong Cats and Adelaide Crows AFL teams.

He was a senior Team Leader for the provision of medical services at the 2000 Sydney Olympic Games and has taught on medical courses conducted by the International Olympic Committee.

His medical practice is devoted to helping all patients – regardless of age or ability – to stay active and 'age youthfully' by adopting his healthy living advice and lifestyle habits.

In more recent years he has also focused on community and population health by delivering messages on healthy lifestyle to all individuals. He is passionate about promoting healthy living for all to improve quality of life, longevity and to reduce health care costs in the Australian community. He believes many of the lessons learnt from dealing with elite sport performance can be applied to everyday productivity and success in the workplace and in life in general.

Peter is regularly seen and heard on television and radio on current affairs, news and lifestyle programs in his role as a media commentator and spokesperson on health and fitness topics. He has become known for his sharp wit, ability to read the play and make complex medical concepts easy for listeners to understand. It was here where he adopted the now infamous name, 'Doc Larkins'.

In his spare time he enjoys good wine, good food, good company and good books. He exercises for health and to help justify the wine and food.

Acknowledgements

Writing this book involved many stages. It would never have reached publication without the support, inspiration, guidance, and feedback from some amazing and loyal individuals.

I want to acknowledge my mum and dad, Cecilia, and Frank, for allowing me to pursue my life goals inspired by their values and dedication. My two sisters Maureen and Noeleen, and my brother Frank, for nurturing the value of family.

My sons, Thomas, Charlie, and Jeremy — this is for you, with love.

Jaynie, you supported me through the difficult times and are a constant positive light even when distracted by life's hurdles. You know what that means to me. #jaypal.

To Bob Talbot, who kept telling me 'Write the Book!' Here it is Bob!

To Sharyn, who is a true confidante and rock of support over so many years and challenges.

To John Di Natale, who encouraged, listened, provided ideas, and gave initial structure advice over many weekend coffees in our village.

To Coral Brown, for your wisdom, and calm influence, also over many coffees!

To Julie Stafford, herself a star author, who's done it before but was generous and challenging with her ideas, feedback and nudges to keep going.

To my Wiley team — who would have thought it would take so many of you to get this book out there!? To Lucy Raymond who took a punt on a first-time author (thank you), Leigh McLennon, Charlotte Duff (who wasn't too brutal at editing out some of my favourite bits!), Chris Shorten and Ingrid Bond, the graphics and copy-editing team, and Renee Aurish in marketing — all of whom contributed to the final product.

To all my closest friends, many of whom shared the journey with me and understood the task — but especially to Geoff, Sandy, Michael and De, my other 'family', who are my constant supporters.

And finally … to Antonia, my much loved and trusted friend, PA, colleague and world class transcriber, feedback expert and critic. There are so many things in my life that you have shared and would not have happened without your kindness and care — this book is merely one of them.

Introduction

Why did I decide to write this book? To be perfectly honest, I have been asking myself the same question repeatedly ever since the idea for this project came to mind back in 2018.

Since then, I have been motivated by comments from my closest friends and some of my patients with whom I shared the idea for writing a book. When I told them the title, I received nothing short of encouragement from each and every one of the select few I told. Subsequently, when I mentioned I had started writing my book, and gave some details of the stages I had achieved, the encouragement was even more forthcoming. The finished product has taken some time, but I needed to make sure it covered all the messages and lifestyle strategies I wanted to discuss before it was published.

So, what do I know about health, healthy living, aging (or, more correctly, 'anti-aging') and longevity? I guess the real answer to that question starts with my early development years and my longstanding interest in physical activity and performance.

A bit about me

My sporting career began with my participation as a very young athlete in Little Athletics (LA) in Geelong. (Geelong was my hometown and where LA began in 1962.) My athletics involvement not only allowed me to appreciate fitness but also motivated me to study which types of exercise and fitness activities gave me the greatest performance return. It also sparked my interest in topics such as nutrition, sleep, training and recovery — all from the ripe old age of six years! LA was my first love as a sport, and I have the distinction of being the first male athlete to compete and graduate through the LA system and subsequently be selected in an Australian Olympic track and field team, in 1976 for the Montreal Olympic Games. (Debbie Wells from NSW, a talented teenage sprinter and teammate, was the first female).

My interest in the field of fitness and performance continued to flourish throughout my athletics career, medical training, and many years in private medical practice in the field of sports and exercise medicine. I have continued to learn and develop my expertise, and have remained curious about how to achieve high performance in life rather than purely in the athletic arena. In this book, I've included some of my personal experiences as an athlete, junior doctor and now a more senior specialist sports and exercise physician. Hopefully the anecdotes and life experiences add to the information provided and help you apply it to your own situation.

While I have had a longstanding involvement in the world of elite sport and sports performance, my current interest in optimal life performance was sparked back in 2005, when I was approached by the Melbourne City Council to provide a presentation on the topic of 'work–life balance'. Ironically, this was not a term I was familiar with. After doing some background research, I was surprised to find quite a lot of interest and research in this field, albeit rudimentary and in its infancy at that stage. Within this theme of work–life balance, the focus for my presentation to Melbourne City Council employees and administration was how physical activity could be integrated into each work week. I spoke to the audience about the health benefits of exercise, which were well researched, particularly in relation to cardiovascular disease prevention, and how to create some personal 'self-time'. Even then, I was encouraging my audience to take responsibility for their life health journey and to increase physical activity as a lifelong health-promoting habit.

Over subsequent years, I have presented this seminar in dozens of different formats, and the content has evolved dramatically. I've also developed gender-specific content, looking at the issues faced by men and women, particularly as they age, and their related health needs. However, my core messages have been consistent throughout that time — that is, my conviction about the beneficial role of physical activity and exercise in personal health protection, and the need for all people, regardless of age, to take control of their lifestyle habits and assume responsibility for looking after themselves.

Far too often over my many years of experience, I've seen people, including those in my profession, blindly accept declines in physical performance, enjoyment and overall lifestyle as a supposedly 'inevitable' consequence of the clock progressing. I've seen way too many individuals take a passive approach to health maintenance and then expect the medical profession to 'fix' the problems after they arise. This is not a sustainable attitude, and I've written this book to challenge some of those myths and concepts. Good habits need to be developed, ideally at an early age, but really at any age to minimise the oft-labelled 'inevitable' effects of aging.

Ultimately, I've written this book to help you work on your healthy lifestyle choices so you can be the best you can be, for as long as you can be.

What this book will do for you

Throughout my many years working in the medical, health and fitness industry, my goal has always been to help my patients and clients to achieve their optimal performance in life — whether they are involved in competitive sport or recreational exercise, or simply trying to be the best they can be in their overall life journey and career. I have also worked to apply the knowledge I have gained working in high-performance sport and translate this into achieving high performance in everyday life. In my time, I have achieved great satisfaction from assisting individuals to improve their lifestyle, fitness and health, and to achieve a higher level of functioning than they previously had.

I'm hoping that by reading this book, you will also embark on the same journey and ultimate achievement.

In the following chapters, I've provided lifestyle tips and habits designed to improve your wellbeing and health, and enhance your prospects of living a long and productive life. My focus is not simply about improving your longevity; I also want to help you improve your quality of life, now and in the future, and be your most productive self — in your personal life and in your career.

I've included scientific facts and the latest medical research, mixed in with my personal experience and some humour. Most importantly, the information included here is intended to offset the all too frequent acceptance of what many see as 'aging changes'. I have always known there is no magic 'fountain of youth' and my research for this book confirms that. However, the messages contained here give you the ingredients to optimise your youthfulness, physically and mentally, as you gracefully age towards 100 years and beyond.

Some sections of this book are more straightforward and factual; in other sections I become more philosophical, as I reflect on things

I would like to have done better. My life has not been smooth and is far from perfect. I have faced many setbacks, the majority of them personal and, in some cases, brought about through my own misguided or naïve decisions, at least in some part. I believe I am my greatest critic and the person I have disappointed most in life is myself. As with everyone, my journey continues.

In this book, I pass on the wisdom and tips I have gained, not because I want to be an evangelist or preacher, but simply to let you know that life is a continuing journey of lessons learned. I'm continuing to try to improve myself and be the best version of myself. I attempt to do the best job I can, albeit far from a perfect performance, for me, my children, my closest friends and all those whom I deal with in life. I hope this book helps you do the same.

How to use this book

The Healthy Hundred is all about giving you choices. After a quick outline of the current state of health in Australia in part I, I then cover in part II common chronic health issues — and how you can avoid them or reduce their impacts. Then, in part III, I outline many (specifically, 100!) actions you can take to improve your optimal performance and healthspan, and live a healthier, happier and longer life.

I've organised the 100 actions in part III under five key themes that, based on my research and personal life experience, I believe help you achieve the goal of living to a healthy 100 years and beyond. These themes are:

1. *Exercise:* Focusing on the role of physical activity as your best health habit and supplement.

2. *Nutrition:* Understanding the importance of healthy eating.

3. *Habits:* Considering how your lifestyle choices and behaviour practices affect your health.

4. *Mindset:* Developing your own healthy perspective on life.

5. *Connection:* Looking at the critical role friendships and social relationships and connectivity play in healthy life balance.

You don't need to adopt every action immediately, and you don't have to read the book cover to cover before getting started. Perhaps after reading parts I and II, you'll scan through the 100 ways outlined in part III and choose a mixture of options to commence your health journey. You can always choose more as you progress.

Also keep in mind that this book is not meant to be a substitute for professional medical care. This is not a medical textbook; the medical advice is general in nature and is intended to help you improve your lifestyle behaviours and to initiate conversations with your preferred treating doctor. If you have any concerns in relation to your own medical care or individual conditions, these should be addressed with your family medical advisor.

While the potential for living to 100 years and beyond is now a reality in our current society, it is more important that you remain healthy, productive and energetic during the remaining years you have in life, regardless of the number you achieve. Nevertheless, I want you to set yourself a target of leading a longer, healthier and more productive life, and realise that achieving a healthy and vivacious 100 years of age — and beyond — is a realistic goal if you maintain a healthy lifestyle. By adopting the actions and habits outlined in this book, I hope you will feel that you can gain a healthier, more productive and happier lifestyle in the years ahead.

So let's get started!

PART I
Taking a pulse check on aging and good health

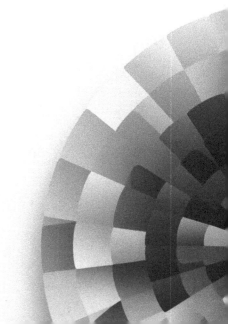

Today, as a society, we seem to be obsessed with staying young. But before we look at how you might slow the aging process, it helps to have a basic understanding of what that process is and what happens to your body as you age. So in this part, I explain some of the reasons we slow down as we grow older—focusing in at a cellular level—and look at some of the illnesses that impede our productivity and function in later life.

Because when people say they want to stay young or don't want to grow old, I think what most are really concerned about is being able to stay active, fit and healthy for as long as they can, and continuing to live their life without disease or limiting disability. That's why in this part, I also introduce you to the idea of healthspan. This is where you move beyond simply extending your life to improving the quality and productivity of that longer life—so you can enjoy those extra years. I also look at the major determinants of good health, and just how many people in Australia are living with ill health. Finally, I tackle whose responsibility it really is to look after your health. (Spoiler alert: it's yours!)

1

Moving from aging to healthspan

In some ways the question 'Why do we age?' might be the most difficult of all to answer. Nevertheless, it really goes to the core of my focus of understanding healthy longevity and ways to slow the aging process. This topic of why we age is broad, with a lot of complicated science behind it. In this chapter, I keep it pretty simple and provide a quick overview of the aging process on a cellular level. I also look at the top reasons Australians die, noting the leading causes for men and women. I then move on to what 'healthy' might mean for you — and how you can improve not only your lifespan but also your healthspan.

Understanding why we age — and die

No doubt you've recognised the signs of aging in someone you know. The external indicators might be greying hair, wrinkled skin, eyesight failure and changes in body posture. These external indicators are generally pretty obvious to others. Some internal shifts, such as cognitive or attitudinal changes, may also be recognised by friends and relatives dealing with an aging individual. Other internal changes might be more obvious to the aging individual, and involve changes to bodily functions (or dysfunctions) — which may be too personal to mention here!

When it comes to causes of death, how frequently do we hear the simple explanation that someone died from 'old age'? Another term often used to explain a death is 'natural causes'. What exactly does this mean? It is far easier to understand the reasons when someone passes away from a cardiac event, cancer or other recognised medical condition, rather than simply from 'old age'.

Focusing in on our cells

Since the 1960s, molecular scientists have studied the decline in function of the body's cellular structures and processes as it ages. (The gradual failure of cell health is referred to as 'senescence' — literally, 'aging failure'.) This area of science, known as 'geroscience', looks at ways to prevent, delay or potentially reverse the aging hallmarks, particularly those caused by chronic diseases.

As we age, the body accumulates senescent, or damaged, cells more rapidly in our aging years. Senescent cells are associated with damage to heart and brain tissue, as well as the inhibition of lung and bone metabolism. The capacity to repair, excrete or reduce the number of these senescent cells is an individual thing, but promising evidence suggests that regular physical activity and exercise promotes the clearance of these damaged senescent cells, and this clearance process can delay the chronic aging symptoms. In many animal studies, for example, exercise has been associated with increased clearance of these cells and hence the link to anti-aging changes in our key body systems. In other words, adopt these habits in your lifestyle and you can age more slowly. Now we are talking progress!

What about our DNA (deoxyribonucleic acid)? DNA is the self-replicating material present in all our chromosomes and carries our unique genetic material. The health of our DNA is critical as we age, and our chromosomes are protected at their ends by structures known as telomeres. Telomeres inhibit damage to our chromosomes, but they deteriorate and become shorter as we age. Some studies suggest that regular physical activity can delay these telomere changes and hence lead to more effective chromosome protection.

Within the cells, mitochondria also play an important role in our health systems, and their function also declines with age because of senescent damage. Again, exercise has been associated with a reduction in this damaging process. (I discuss mitochondrial function in more detail in chapter 6.)

Finally, aging has been associated with increased accumulation of inflammatory markers in the body. Aging processes can be slowed down by interventions that reduce these inflammatory markers and assist with metabolism and limiting the damage related to everyday oxidative processes. One of the key interventions, again, is exercise. Can you see the recurring theme here?

This overview highlights that aging is a multifactorial process generally associated with a decline in our cell function because of many everyday body processes. While more research is certainly needed, there are encouraging signs to show the role of physical activity and regular exercise in delaying and potentially reversing these aging processes resulting from cell damage.

So, why do we die?

Death is a complex topic but, within the focus of this book, I've included here some statistics on what we know about why we are all mortal!

According to the federal government's Australian Institute of Health and Welfare, the leading causes of male deaths in Australia in 2020 were as follows:

1. coronary artery disease

2. dementia (including Alzheimer's disease)

3. lung cancer

4. cerebrovascular disease (for example, stroke)

5. prostate cancer

6. chronic obstructive pulmonary disease

7. diabetes

8. colorectal (bowel) cancer

9. suicide

10. accidental falls.

For females, the leading causes of death were:

1. dementia (including Alzheimer's disease)

2. coronary artery disease

3. cerebrovascular disease

4. lung cancer

5. breast cancer

6. chronic obstructive pulmonary disease

7. colorectal (bowel) cancer

8. diabetes

9. heart failure complications

10. accidental falls.

You might be surprised that dementia and Alzheimer's disease rank so highly as leading causes of death in both men and women. I suspect many of the other causes will be familiar. Most are discussed in the following pages. (For more information and helpful resources from the Australian Institute of Health and Welfare, go to www .aihw.gov.au.)

Why aim for 100 and beyond? The Queen's telegram!

I must admit, when I was a youngster growing up, I was not aware of the concept of longevity. When you are a child, you mostly live in the present and don't have much concept of the future. However, one thing I was aware of was that I had many relatives who appeared to me as being 'really old'. One of the other traditions that I became aware of at a relatively young age was that when someone turned 100 years of age, they received a telegram from Her Majesty Queen Elizabeth II in England. In other words, reaching 100 years was considered such an achievement that even the Queen of England would acknowledge it! To me, that seemed an outstanding achievement in 'life years'.

However, as you will see in the chapters of this book, many people are now living to 100 — and beyond — in modern society. In fact, the World Economic Forum has estimated that in 2022 around 573,000 individuals were over 100 years old. It is no longer the novelty that I thought it was. So my intention with

(continued)

writing this book is to provide you with the information and materials to become someone who not only receives the traditional telegram (or is it an email from King Charles these days?!), but also can aim to live beyond 100 years, just as many of the inhabitants of certain regions of the world with the longest living populations have already shown is possible. (These regions are known as 'blue zones' and I discuss them in in chapter 10.)

Working out what 'healthy' means

I must admit that over the many years that I have been working in the health and fitness industry, I have had to adjust my attitudes to what constitutes a healthy living program. In my early days, I probably oversimplified things, thinking that a good mixture of exercise with 'healthy, balanced eating' was sufficient to provide health and longevity. It was a formula that was easy to preach, but over time I have realised many other components need to be integrated into a more complete healthy lifestyle.

While exercise and healthy eating are certainly essential, I have learned and accepted, particularly in more recent times, that many other factors can also boost your anti-aging, health-promoting prospects. Diverse aspects such as social connectivity, mindset, family, personal development and even the role of mentors all contribute to nurturing a healthy, long life, and I cover these over the course of this book. While no 'one size fits all' recipe for health exists, it is important that the core factors are addressed and that you learn which individual ones apply best to your metabolism, genetics and lifestyle.

This process obviously can take some time and may involve a period of trial and error before determining the best fit for you. Ultimately, some experience and then consistent application of the correct balance of these lifestyle factors is required to achieve the long and healthy life you seek. (That's the ex-athlete coming out in me. Steady consistent training and looking after your body's health equals best performance results!)

What is a healthy lifestyle?

So, what are the core health factors, and what constitutes a healthy lifestyle? Several components go into the blend, but generally a healthy lifestyle can be summarised in the following:

1. behaviour choices that promote wellbeing

2. regular physical activity and exercise

3. healthy nutrition

4. optimal sleep

5. social integration and connectivity

6. a healthy mindset with emotional stability

7. a positive environment in which to live and work

8. lack of dangerous risk taking

9. work–life harmony

10. time for self—prioritising wellbeing.

This book will address all of these (and more) in the coming chapters as I outline my healthy lifestyle tips. Some tips are quite specific, while others are more general and able to be interpreted or introduced depending on your individual circumstances and current health situation.

Focusing on your healthspan

In my earlier days when I was promoting the value of exercise and healthy living practices, I believed that the end goal was to live a *healthier*, more fruitful life through these good practices—my focus was all about quality, rather than duration (quantity). Of course, at that time, I hoped that by looking after themselves and minimising illness risk, my patients and clients (and the audiences I was presenting to) would also live a *longer* life. However, this hope was not yet supported by a great deal of high-quality validated research. So I focused on what was supported, and regularly used to say, 'Exercise may not make you live a day longer, but you will live a longer day.'

My message then was clear—being fit and healthy allows you to be more productive in your day and get the most out of what you do. Whether you lived a longer time to do exactly that was controversial and often disputed by others in my field. At that time, research was more focused on the value of exercise in the management of and recovery from cardiac problems such as heart attacks due to ischaemic heart disease. The positive impact of exercise on conditions such as diabetes, stroke, cancers and mental health was not yet appreciated by most in the medical and other allied health professions.

Since that time, literally hundreds of validated scientific studies have been published which confirm that regular physical activity and healthy living choices do result in an individual living longer and with better quality of life in their later years. The logic is obvious—if you are not unwell and do not die prematurely from preventable diseases, you will live longer. However, what is more important than simple longevity (long life) is the concept now known as 'healthspan'. Healthspan is defined as the period of life spent in good health, free from the chronic diseases and disabilities of aging. Importantly, the concept focuses in on the number of *disease-free years* people enjoy towards the end of their lifespan. In other words, focusing on your healthspan helps you live longer (quantity) *and* be healthier and more productive (quality) in your later years. What a deal!

TIP

By understanding what healthspan means to you and considering the quality of life you'd like to enjoy as you age, you can start to focus in on what lifestyle changes you might need to make.

Key takeaways

Many destructive metabolic processes are occurring every day in your body. These have a negative impact on cell health, performance and longevity. Ultimately, you age faster if these destructive processes go unchecked. How you live, what you eat, whether you exercise and how you look after yourself overall can positively influence your individual aging process. You do have control over these processes.

2

Your health: Whose responsibility is it?

In my medical experience, far too many individuals take a passive approach to health maintenance. They look for 'someone else' to ensure they stay healthy—usually their chosen medical practitioner. My recurring message in this book is that you need to take a positive and active role in promoting your own health situation. Good health is not a given right that you acquire passively.

The medical information supporting health promotion is well established and generally consistent. While I understand advice can at times seem contradictory, this book is all about cutting through any confusion and providing clear ways to take control of your own health.

If you are one of those people who feel that your good health is something that should come naturally, you need to reconsider your position. In this chapter, I run through some of the factors that influence good health, the types of chronic illnesses reported by many Australians, and how you can start to take charge and actively improve your health.

Understanding what determines good health

Three broad categories can influence your good health outcomes throughout your life: genetics, environment and behaviour. While you might not be able to do much about your genetics, you'll discover throughout this book the many ways you can adjust your environment and your behaviour for positive health benefits.

Genetics

Clearly your DNA can influence your health profile. Certain families, for example, have a higher incidence of medical conditions such as breast cancer, bowel cancer or heart disease. These conditions are passed from generation to generation, sometimes skipping one generation, but then appearing again. This highlights the importance of knowing your family background and having regular testing for any known high-risk conditions in your genetics.

While your DNA is one particular risk determinant that can be difficult to influence, keep in mind that in more recent times the role of genetics has been challenged. Genetics is currently thought to influence only 20 to 25 per cent of our health and illness risk. The majority is influenced by other factors, particularly lifestyle choices. Read on!

Environment

Many health conditions are influenced by both the domestic residential and occupational environment in which you function. People who live in cities with bad air pollution, poor water quality and toxic chemicals associated with waste product emissions can be at risk of conditions such as chronic respiratory disorders (such as asthma, emphysema and obstructive diseases) as well as certain cancers (such as skin, asbestosis and lung).

In developing countries where solid fuel burning is used every day in both cooking and heating, for example, the incidence of chronic respiratory disease is higher than in more developed countries. This clearly affects quality of life and lifespan. (For more information on the impact of environment on health, a great place to start is the World Health Organization — www.who.int.)

Behaviour

This component of health status has been estimated to contribute more than 50 per cent to your quality of life and illness risk. Personal lifestyle choices such as smoking, poor nutrition habits and physical inactivity are all contributing factors here — and they are all factors over which every individual has some control. Changing your behaviour choices allows you to influence your own personal health direction. 'Acquired' health conditions such as obesity, diabetes or the effects of excessive alcohol intake are associated with poor health outcomes and are often synergistic in determining other health risks when combined with other environmental and lifestyle behaviours.

Just how sick is Australia?

Many studies produced annually detail statistics on health and illness in Australia. Whilst the precise numbers often vary, the pattern of illness and the most common conditions remain consistent.

One of the most reliable sources—the Australian Bureau of Statistics—released the following health information from the 2021 census:

- Over 8 million people reported having a long-term health condition (or 31.7 per cent of the population)

- 4.8 million people had one of the selected long-term health conditions.

- 1.5 million people had two of the selected long-term health conditions.

- 772 000 people had three or more of the selected long-term health conditions.

The types of chronic health conditions listed in the 2021 census for self-selection were:

- heart disease

- diabetes

- mental health condition

- arthritis

- asthma

- dementia

- cancer

- lung condition

- stroke

- kidney disease

- other.

Of course, coming from the census means that this health data is self-reported, but nevertheless the numbers are alarming. Almost one-third of people in the Australian community report they are living with and attempting to manage a chronic health condition. The economic impact of this is clearly crippling for the federal and state governments — in 2022–23 alone, the federal government's total spending on 'health' was $106 billion (up from $100 billion the previous year). And this figure doesn't include money spent by other levels of government, individuals and other non-government funders, such as private health insurers. In my mind, the way the healthcare system functions is 'back to front', with the expenditure really being directed at illness care.

Surely it is better to spend money on prevention and education on minimising or eliminating these afflictions rather than continuing to have huge funding costs related to treating these conditions in our overburdened healthcare system?

Working out what you need to do

This is where the onus falls back on the individual to seek appropriate advice on their respective health profile and to assess the obvious measurable factors. YOU have to take action! You're never too old and it's never too late to make healthy lifestyle changes. This includes knowing your blood pressure, cholesterol (lipids) and blood sugar levels as well as seeking advice on your nutrition and exercise profile and weight management program.

Too many individuals have a 'fix it once it's broken' attitude. As a nation, we spend over $23 billion per annum on pharmaceutical medications to treat illness. Over 100 million prescriptions for cardiovascular medications are written annually. We seek out pills to treat blood pressure, high cholesterol, diabetes, obesity, insomnia and mental health conditions. Massive government healthcare budgets include costs associated with sophisticated treatments for heart disease and cancers. These treatments are, of course, important in the community; unfortunately, however, the conditions are often detected late and require lengthy and difficult treatment protocols.

What if a single non-pharmaceutical product had a positive influence on virtually all the known medical conditions and chronic illnesses, as well as a positive benefit on risk factor reduction? What if this product was free?

This 'product' is currently available and has been verified by decades of randomly controlled scientific studies to validate its benefits. It's not a pill — the 'product' is called *physical activity*. That's right, exercise is medicine. As Greek philosopher Socrates argued centuries ago, 'Is not the bodily habit spoiled by rest and idleness, but preserved for a long time by motion and exercise?'

Science has now caught up with philosophy. Since the early 20th century, studies have been documenting the value of physical activity and exercise in reducing common morbidities such heart disease, diabetes and blood pressure. With the advent of more sophisticated and rigorous research techniques, these results have been reproduced consistently — and yet the message is still not well heard by the community.

More recent scientific studies have shown that a mixture of aerobic (cardiovascular) activity and some regular strength training has a positive benefit on heart disease, diabetes, blood pressure, mental health and obesity. And one of the most exciting advances I have seen in my time working in the discipline of exercise medicine has been the emergence of validated studies that show the incidence, response to treatment and recurrence rate of many common cancers are all positively enhanced by patients who engage in regular physical activity. These studies have been undertaken for breast cancer, bowel cancer, prostate cancer and lung cancer. Many other studies are pending which I anticipate will reinforce these findings.

A clear message also is that you do not need to be training like an athlete to get these exercise-related benefits. You only need to do activity at a low to moderate level to have a positive impact on your health. In fact, the biggest gain occurs when people change from doing absolutely nothing to as little as 60 minutes of (predominantly aerobic) activity per week. Studies have shown this simple change can achieve the largest gain of a 25 per cent reduction in all causes of death. No drug in the world has that impact across so many health conditions! Of course, additional benefits emerge as you move to some higher levels of exercise per week, with the ultimate 'sweet spot' being around 150 minutes per week. Other studies have shown individuals who consistently exercise in the range of 150 to 200 minutes per week have been shown to have up to a 40 per cent reduction in mortality risk for the most common illness conditions.

I cover incorporating exercise into your lifestyle in much more detail in chapter 6, including the importance of undergoing a health check prior to beginning a physical activity program, particularly if you have been inactive for many years and are currently being treated for existing medical conditions.

TIP
Exercise is medicine — and its potential benefits are amazing!

Key takeaways

Healthy longevity is not just about good genetics, and is instead a complex blend of many components and behaviours. The important thing to keep in mind when considering factors that influence your health is that you have more influence and control over your health than you realise.

While regular health check-ups are essential, the ultimate prescription your doctor should be providing includes undertaking a regular physical activity program—which will help you keep away from your doctor's office! The level of exercise does not need to be intensive in the beginning but can gradually increase to provide more fitness benefits as time goes by. You can't take any short cuts in this process, but the results are cumulative and consistent. You just have to move!

PART II
Monitoring your health

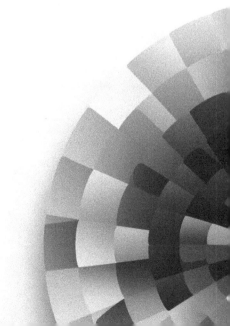

No doubt you already have some awareness of, and indeed experience of, chronic illness and disease — either through friends, family or work colleagues, or even potentially through your own experience. These experiences are extremely hard to live through; however, generally a lesson can be learnt from any unfortunate illness event. Understanding the background to these illnesses can assist in future reduction of their impact.

In the next few chapters, I outline the most common chronic (and killer) illnesses, and suggest strategies to detect and minimise the negative impact they have on your health and longevity. I also offer some gender-specific information — because, yes, men and women are different! —busting the macho myths about 'sucking it up' and waiting until something breaks before you try to fix it. Finally, I run through the importance of regular health check-ups, because regular monitoring of physical and mental health is important for everyone, and can help prevent more serious illnesses down the track.

3

Key medical conditions to understand — and avoid

As covered in the previous chapter, 8 million people in Australia (almost one-third) report they are living with a long-term health condition such as heart disease, diabetes or a mental health condition. That's a staggering number of people living with a chronic illness that reduces their ability to enjoy and participate in life, every day. Of course, funding and care needs to be in place to help these people. However, we all also need to be focused on education and prevention — being aware of the warning signs and how to avoid these chronic problems.

That's what this chapter is all about. I outline the common chronic illnesses and debilitating conditions in Australia, and how you can take charge of your own health and do what you can to avoid them.

Keeping your heart healthy

Unfortunately, cardiovascular disease and heart illness are the number one causes of morbidity and death in Australia. In 2021, over 17 000 acute coronary deaths occurred in Australia from myocardial infarction (heart attack). If you include all types of heart attacks, strokes and arrhythmia, cardiovascular problems contributed to 42 348 deaths. Both men and women are at risk and the gender gap has become smaller over the last decade.

Heart disease is also the number one budget spend on illness care in our nation. In 2019, we saw over 519 000 hospital admissions for cardiac disease treatment. Experts estimate that in individuals aged 25 and over, more than 160 acute coronary episodes of heart attack occur every day. This incidence of sudden death is still way too common, especially when access to acute medical care is lacking or delayed. The role of defibrillators remains essential in the ability to save lives.

What are the potential signs of a heart problem? The following are signs the heart is the likely cause of an impending problem:

- chest pain — either with exercise or at rest

- chest tightness or chest pressure

- jaw, shoulder, arm pain or aching or heaviness in the left side of the body

- breathlessness

- pulse irregularity — fast or missed beats

- cough — accumulation of lung fluid (indicating congestive heart failure)

- unusual fatigue

- reduced exercise capacity

- dizziness or light-headedness

- 'heart burn'—frequent use of indigestive medicines (antacids).

If you recognise any of these symptoms, book yourself in for a thorough check with your GP to identify any early symptoms and either exclude heart problems or have them further investigated. This check will include:

- a detailed history of the symptoms and circumstances provoking them

- examination of heart sounds, lungs and blood pressure

- a test for your blood lipids (cholesterol), insulin and inflammation markers

- potentially a CT angiogram (CTA), which will report a calcium score, indicative of plaque deposits in the main heart arteries

- perhaps an exercise echocardiogram—a functional test under exercise load to watch the heart perform

- sometimes a more traditional angiogram image of the blood vessels

- other more sophisticated targeted tests as warranted by the earlier findings.

Remember—your heart is one of the critical organs of your body and needs to be kept healthy throughout your lifetime. All the messages and tips throughout this book contribute to overall health and in particular heart health. Make sure you look after yours.

Avoiding strokes

A stroke occurs when a blood vessel in the brain suddenly becomes blocked, ruptures or begins to bleed. A stroke is frequently fatal, but advances in diagnosis, detection and medical care have dramatically improved survival rates. Along with cardiac events, stroke is considered a condition related to the cardiovascular system (CVS), and these two conditions combine to become the number one cause of death in Australia (and worldwide).

Precise data on stroke incidence in Australia is not as well documented as other medical conditions such as heart attacks and cancers. However, according to 2021 data from the Australian Institute of Health and Welfare (AIHW), around 387 000 Australians aged 50 and over (1.3 per cent of our population) have experienced a stroke at some stage in their lives. Self-reported data from the Australian Bureau of Statistics in 2019 supported this figure.

Stroke is more common in older age groups, with 71 per cent of people who reported incidents being over 75 years. Strokes occur more frequently with advancing age and the highest proportion is in those over 85 years. This is true for both men and women.

In 2018, experts estimated 38 600 stroke events occurred in Australia — more than 100 every day. According to the Australia Stroke Foundation, someone in Australia experiences a stroke every 19 minutes. The incidence of stroke events declined slightly over the past 20 years, but since 2013 rates have levelled out for both men and women. They are a common cause of hospitalisations, and in 2019 stroke was believed to be the underlying cause of 8400 deaths in Australia (5 per cent of all deaths). This still means it is one of the leading causes of death in Australia. As a cause of death, it is more potent than prostate cancer in men and breast cancer in women. Its impact on the economic health budget is substantial with both direct and indirect costs estimated at over $32 billion.

While many causes of stroke are related to the presence of an aneurysm (a localised expansion and weakness in a brain blood vessel), it can be difficult to detect these until the bleeding incident occurs. However, advances in acute neurosurgical medical care, including clot retrieval from the brain, have vastly improved survival rates. The Stroke Foundation reports that almost half a million Australians are living with the after-effects of a stroke.

A milder form of stroke is known as a 'transient ischaemic attack' (TIA). A TIA is a temporary blockage of the blood supply to a part of the brain which may only last for a few minutes, but produces stroke-like symptoms such as confusion, weakness, slurred speech or loss of balance. Fortunately, a TIA usually causes no permanent damage to the brain. However, people who have experienced a TIA have been shown to be at a much higher risk of a future stroke.

The good news is that strokes are preventable, and your risk is affected by lifestyle. Diseases of the blood vessels due to arthrosclerosis and plaque (such as ischaemic heart disease in the heart blood vessels) are the most likely causes and can be due to the lifestyle factors discussed elsewhere in this book. Exercise together with healthy eating and maintaining a healthy weight are important in promoting good blood vessel health. Screening for high-risk cardiovascular disorders including regular health check-ups, blood tests and lifestyle advice are also important preventive measures. Regular brain scans to check for the presence of aneurysms are not recommended because this is an expensive investigation and the yield is not likely to be justified on a risk–benefit financial basis.

The Stroke Foundation has developed the FAST test as an easy way to recognise and remember the signs of a developing stroke. These are:

- *Face:* Check the face. Has the mouth dropped?

- *Arms:* Can the arms be lifted?

- *Speech:* Is speech slurred? Can the person understand you?

- *Time:* Time is critical.

If any of these signs are present, call emergency services immediately (000).

TIP

With a stroke, rapid recognition = rapid treatment = better survival and recovery.

For further help with minimising your risk of stroke, follow the health guidelines throughout this book.

Protecting your lungs

I suspect I do not need to explain how important the lungs are in keeping you healthy. Lungs are the critical organs that convert the air you breathe into oxygen in your bloodstream and hence give you the ability to perform your everyday functions. Without your lungs, you simply can't live. (Apologies to the heart and brain for this statement.)

Out of all deaths caused by cancer, death due to lung cancer remains number one. Bowel cancer is number two. AIHW cancer data estimates 14 529 new lung cancer diagnoses in 2022, with males slightly in the dominant group. This represents 9 per cent of all new cancer diagnoses. Experts also estimate approximately 8664 deaths were caused by lung cancer in 2022, with 4855 in males and 3809 in females. This represents 17 per cent of all deaths from cancer in Australia.

The five-year survival of lung cancer is around 22 per cent of individuals, not an encouraging statistic. Survival depends on the stage of diagnosis, the type of cancer and the overall health of the individual. Reviewing the trends over the last decade or so, it appears that the number of new cases of lung cancer is gradually reducing as fewer people are smoking and awareness of healthy lifestyle choices is increasing. Lung cancer deaths tend to be in people who have been smokers in their 'previous lives', particularly in the critical decades of the 20s, 30s and 40s age groups.

According to Cancer Australia, tobacco remains the single largest cause of lung cancer globally. It reports that 90 per cent of Australian men and 65 per cent of Australian women who die from lung cancer are tobacco smokers. The only positive news is that the heavy publicity about the dangers of smoking has reduced the overall number of people smoking—smoking prevalence has decreased substantially over the past 30 years and more than 80 per cent of Australian adolescents state that they have never smoked.

Unfortunately, however, according to data recently released by Cancer Council Victoria's Centre for Behavioural Research in Cancer (CBRC), the proportion of teenagers smoking has increased for the first time in 25 years. The study revealed the proportion of 14 to 17 year olds smoking tobacco increased from 2.1 per cent in 2018 to 6.7 per cent in 2022. Vaping in teenagers is also increasing dramatically, going from less than 1 per cent of 14 to 17 year olds in 2018 to 11.8 per cent in 2022 and 14.5 per cent in early 2023.

Experts at CBRC argue vaping can be a gateway into smoking, with studies finding those who vape are three times as likely to take up smoking later. This dangerous trend needs to be reversed if Australia is to continue to see lung cancer gradually declining as a common cause of disability and death in the coming years. (If you need more reasons to quit smoking, see chapter 8.)

Diagnosis of lung cancers is not as simple as some of the other cancer types (such as skin or bowel cancers). While more advanced lung cancers may show up on chest imaging such as an x-ray, it is much more important to pick up the common early symptoms. These include:

- a persistent cough

- coughing up blood stained or coloured sputum

- unusual chest pain

- loss of appetite

- unexplained weight loss

- shortness of breath

- overall lethargy.

Of course, many of these are non-specific symptoms, but the cough or blood-stained sputum should trigger important investigations.

Unfortunately, no reliable blood test is available to detect lung cancer. The final diagnosis is obtained through a tissue biopsy of lung tissue, often via a bronchoscopy, where a tube and camera is placed into the lung bronchial system. By obtaining a sample of any abnormal tissue, what's known as the 'staging' of a lung cancer can be undertaken. (Staging tells you and your healthcare provider about the severity and size of your cancer and whether it has spread.) This analysis then allows for the appropriate introduction of treatments, which may include surgery, chemotherapy, radiotherapy or, more recently, immunotherapy. Immunotherapy is one of the greatest advances in cancer treatments because it harnesses the body's own immune response cells as a way of treating multiple cancer types, including lung, bowel and skin.

Other ways to obtain a tissue diagnosis have been developed, and are particularly useful if the lung tumour is lower down in the lungs and not accessible with a traditional bronchoscopy. Techniques can include a CT guided lung biopsy, endobronchial ultrasound biopsy or perhaps a thoracoscopy, where tissue can be accessed from deeper parts of the lung. These are all quite complex procedures but are regularly undertaken by medical specialists who work in this field.

The message again is simple — if you notice any suspicious signs of any lung dysfunction, including a persistent cough, blood-stained sputum or unexplained lethargy and weight loss, then lung cancer needs to be considered by your doctor as one of the potential diagnoses. Please report any of these symptoms and have yourself checked.

Checking your bowel (colon)

Bowel cancer (also known as colorectal cancer) was the fourth most diagnosed cancer in Australia in 2021. It ranks behind breast cancer, prostate cancer and skin melanoma. As a cause of death from cancer, however, bowel cancer is second only to lung cancer in Australia.

According to the AIHW, 15 540 new cases were diagnosed in 2021 in Australia, with a slight tendency for males to be more affected. This represents 10 per cent of all the new cancer cases diagnosed. The AIHW also outlined that bowel cancer resulted in approximately 5295 known deaths, again with males slightly more at risk. This represents 11 per cent of all the cancer deaths in Australia in 2021.

While the five-year survival rate of bowel cancer is around 70 per cent after diagnosis, the actual result depends on the stage of the cancer at diagnosis and other factors such as the health of the individual and treatment undertaken. The earlier the diagnosis is made through appropriate bowel screening, the more likely that appropriate treatment is instituted, and survival chances can be increased. The Australian federal government provides people over the age of 50 with a free faecal occult blood (FOB) test, which can be undertaken in the privacy of your home. A more detailed test involving colonoscopy of the bowel can also be undertaken on a regular basis to assess for bowel polyps and other pathologies or to detect cancers at an early stage and to institute appropriate treatment. If a colonoscopy detects any abnormal bowel pathology, then regular follow up colonoscopies can be undertaken to monitor the disease.

Diet plays an extremely important role in gut and colon health. High dietary intake of foods containing fibre, such as fruit and vegetables, can protect against many cancers, including bowel cancer. Poor lifestyle choices, on the other hand, such as smoking and excessive consumption of processed meats and fatty red meats, potentially increase the risk of colorectal cancer. To maintain good health and wellbeing the National Health and Medical Research Council (NHMRC) recommends that meat consumption be limited to lean and unprocessed types. Regular exercise has also been proven to be beneficial for reduced incidence of many cancer types, including bowel cancer. (For more on improving your gut health, see chapter 7.)

While we've seen some fantastic advances in the treatment of bowel cancer (and many other cancer conditions) through immunotherapy and improvements in surgical and chemotherapy techniques, it is far more important to prevent this condition. The message is clear — book in for regular check-ups, follow a healthy, unprocessed diet, and get regular exercise. This is another important step in your path to a long healthy life.

Keeping your blood pressure healthy

Most people understand that one important health measure a doctor will assess during a health check-up is your blood pressure. You no doubt will have experienced a blood pressure reading being taken personally — perhaps during a health check-up or time in hospital — or seen it on a multitude of TV shows, often in an accident situation or ambulance scene.

Just what the ideal blood pressure is for any individual can be confusing. When I graduated from medical school, the recommended target for adult blood pressure was a reading of 140mmHg systolic with a reading of 90mmHg diastolic. (The figure is often recorded as 140/90.)

What do these numbers mean?

In the simplest of terms, the 140 'systolic 'refers to the pump pressure the heart is producing in the arteries when it is pushing out blood from its chambers during the maximum pump effort. The 90 'diastolic' (lower figure) refers to the 'resting' pressure within the heart when it is recovering between beats. The lower figure is more important because it reflects the amount of rest the heart muscle is getting between its working beats.

Over time, the recommended levels for ideal blood pressure have varied. It can be confusing when different organisations state different recommended levels for what is a 'normal' or 'ideal' blood pressure. So let's keep it simple. At the time of writing, the recommended 'optimal' figure in Australia for a healthy adult is 120–130/80–85. For children, the figure is generally lower. Anything above 140/90 is noteworthy and should be discussed with your doctor in the context of other lifestyle health indicators such as weight, family history and fitness levels.

Elevated (high) blood pressure (known as 'hypertension') is generally associated with a higher risk of illness, particularly cardiovascular disease, including heart attacks. High blood pressure may be idiopathic (not due to any recognisable cause) or it may be secondary to lifestyle causes, including obesity and lack of fitness. In combination with other risk factors, such as high cholesterol, smoking and poor nutrition, high blood pressure is another factor amplifying the risk of ill health and premature death.

Knowing your average blood pressure is an important health marker. Importantly, blood pressure can vary dramatically during the day, influenced by the time of day, stress, exercise or other activities. During sleep, your blood pressure is generally at its lowest. A single reading of high blood pressure at a doctor's office will not usually be a reason to begin taking blood pressure medication. Raised blood pressure needs to be checked on separate occasions to see if it is consistently high. (High levels in a doctor's office are often referred to as 'white coat hypertension', a reaction to the stress of visiting your doctor! Hopefully you understand your doctor is on your side and a visit shouldn't stress you!)

Another way to get a better indication of your average daily blood pressure is to wear a 24-hour monitor. This device regularly checks your blood pressure during your normal day (or even during a 48-hour period) and gives a more accurate indication of whether you are experiencing high blood pressure or simply an occasional spurt.

High blood pressure rarely produces significant symptoms. It is really one of the silent parameters in your health profile, and this is why it needs to be regularly checked. Very rarely, high blood pressure may cause headaches and these should always be investigated if they are occurring regularly. High blood pressure can also cause a stroke or bleeding in the brain because of the rupture of a weak blood vessel, known as an aneurysm.

Low blood pressure is not as common as hypertension but can also cause problems. It may cause dizziness or loss of balance, especially after rising suddenly from sitting or lying down. Low blood pressure often has no obvious cause, although fatigue, dehydration, excess weight loss or side effects from certain medications need to be ruled out.

The message is simply to keep track of your blood pressure and make sure you are working in the healthy range for your age and fitness level. As with most health conditions covered in this book, regular aerobic exercise provides preventative benefits — in this case, a reduction in blood pressure in most individuals. If you look after yourself, you are far less likely to be one of the thousands of Australians who take blood pressure medication to keep their blood pressure in the normal range. Addressing lifestyle issues is a much better approach.

Staying abreast of your health

No doubt you've already been affected by a family member, colleague, neighbour or acquaintance who has been through the breast cancer process. I've seen it have an impact on many dozens of individuals — not only patients, but also those close to me in my life. Fortunately, many of them are currently managing their breast cancer condition thanks to the treatments they have undergone.

Nevertheless, this has been a challenging process for all and has often involved a range of therapies, including surgery, radiotherapy, chemotherapy (with the traumatic hair loss) and, more recently, immunotherapy. The emotional toll is dramatic. At the time of writing, over 80 000 Australians are estimated to be living with and managing breast cancer. When it occurs in a younger individual, particularly a woman in her 30s, it has a major impact on her family and career. The support network around these people needs to be strong and loving.

Breast cancer was the fifth cause of female deaths in Australians in 2020 and, when the subject of breast disease is raised, most people naturally think of women's health. What many people don't realise is that men can also develop breast tumours and breast cancer conditions. The AIHW estimates that 2022 saw 20 640 new cases of breast cancer in Australia. Of these, the vast majority will be in women; however, over 200 cases will be in males. Of the estimated 3214 breast cancer deaths in 2022, around 36 were in males (1.1 per cent).

Males need to be aware that they can develop an unusual swelling or lump in breast tissue and need to have this checked out quickly by a health practitioner, much the same as a female would do. Overall, females are often much more in tune with their health status from a young age (pretty much from the onset of puberty) and, therefore, can be more alert to these changes. Nevertheless, an unusual lump in male breast tissue, while hopefully benign, may be a cancerous tumour and can be easily assessed with a medical examination followed by imaging and perhaps a tissue biopsy. This is the same process as a female would undergo to investigate a suspicious breast lump.

Breast cancer remains second only to prostate cancer as the most frequently diagnosed cancer in Australia at the time of writing. This reflects better awareness by individuals — leading to them booking in a check-up when they discover a suspicious lump — and better screening. Advances in initial diagnosis and treatment mean that this diagnosis is no longer the daunting and tragic situation it would have been in our parents' and grandparents' time. Between 1989 and 2018, the five-year survival rate of breast cancer improved from 77 per cent to 92 per cent. This is a wonderful advance in the management of breast cancer, but clearly we still have a way to go to get this figure closer to 100 per cent. With the advances in modern treatment, including immunotherapy and better screening, hopefully this will be achieved within the coming years.

While the trend is positive — fewer deaths and longer survival rates — it is important to include breast health checks in your regular health maintenance. For women, this includes regular self-examination and an awareness of the changes that can be expected in breast tissue as part of the normal monthly hormonal cycle. Some thickening and 'lumpiness' within breast tissue, for example, is not unusual over this monthly cycle.

TIP

If you're a woman, the main thing you're looking for when checking your breasts is change. You need to get to know and understand your normal patterns so you can recognise any abnormality such as a lump that does not resolve with the normal cycle time frame. Again, men should also be alert to any changes in their breast tissue.

Breast cancer affects us all. However, it is important that we look at this as a potentially 'curable' disease and take all measures to make sure that cases are identified early. This is another step in maintaining a healthy and long life.

Managing your mental health

In recent years, mental health has become one of the most discussed health topics in society. What was once a relatively 'taboo' topic, smothered in stigma and derided by so many, has now been revealed as a widespread affliction across all age groups. Mental health issues can manifest in so many guises, and their impact on individuals, families, society and the community is widespread.

In the past, our traditional model of health has largely focused on measurable physical parameters. Conditions such as heart disease, stroke, diabetes and cancer have received significant attention and publicity in the battle to promote personal health awareness. These illnesses are still of major importance; however, mental health as another health concern has begun to receive long overdue coverage for the massive impact it has on so many individuals in our community.

In 2014, a study from the Mental Health Commission of NSW reported one in three women and one in four men lived with a mental health condition. Over the almost 10 years since, dozens of public figures — including politicians, athletes, entertainers, first responders, police, community workers, healthcare workers, military and business leaders — have shared their mental health battles. This has certainly helped to promote awareness and encourage many to seek help, but we are a long way from where we need to be.

The reporting and incidence of mental health disorders has risen enormously in recent years. Many reasons have been suggested for this — including previous underreporting, stress from modern lifestyle pressures, social media use, and societal and family changes. The number of very young children experiencing mental health disorders is particularly alarming, with some experts estimating up to 25 per cent of school-age children are affected. In addition, since 2019 the role that the COVID-19 pandemic has played is well documented.

The publicity surrounding community mental health messages has changed a lot in recent years. The focus on mental and emotional health is now headline news in so many areas of our society. Mental illness has always carried a stigma (and probably still does in many areas), but we need to move away from this and understand the importance of this topic and the devastating impact it can have on individual health and society overall. Experts estimate that as many as 20 per cent of the population are undergoing mental health treatment at any given time. The incidence is higher in Australia's First Nations communities.

What is clear is that support for these individuals must be readily available and a long-term management plan put in place to help deal with their condition. Traditional medical intervention—involving counselling and medication via psychological and psychiatric services—is usually required, but a strategy of self-help techniques always forms a component of the treatment pathway.

If you're facing mental health issues, being able to discuss your problems with a trusted friend, colleague or family member is vital. Equally, seeking professional help is important and the promotion of support services has never been as prominent as they are now. Nevertheless, resources remain stretched and waiting times for professional medical advice can still be frustratingly lengthy.

The physical health benefits of investing time in personal wellness promotion have always been known. The mental health benefits are equally well established. (As Greek philosopher Epicurus argued centuries ago, 'The ultimate goal of the blessed life is physical health and mental serenity.')

For decades, studies of people with depression and anxiety have shown positive benefits in mental wellbeing from regular exercise performed for as little as one hour per week. Patients report less anxiety, better sleep and reduced use of medication through participating in light to moderate physical activity. The benefits seem enhanced if the activity is undertaken with a friend or group.

Another dimension to personal health is also important here — your 'sense of self', which reflects your inherent values. This is influential in how you function as an individual and your ability to be a valued co-worker, parent, partner, good mate or trusted colleague. It is an essential component of what is referred to as 'inner (holistic) health'.

In recent surveys of workplace satisfaction and wellbeing, the factors most frequently reported as being concerns to workers were stress, anxiety and depression. This discovery was across both genders and reflects how common these issues are in everyday life. Conditions such as high blood pressure, cholesterol or diabetes were much lower down the list of workers' concerns. I particularly loved the finding that the most valued workplace services were onsite physical activity opportunities, in-house education sessions, walking groups and the availability of quality healthy food. I wish more companies would provide these as a matter of course. If you are the company boss, then get on to it!

You must not take good health, including emotional health, for granted. Making some simple changes to activity levels and lifestyle can have a significant impact and contribute both to longevity and quality of life. See your family doctor or other qualified health care adviser if you recognise the need to discuss mental health issues. Share your concerns with a trusted friend. The stigma needs to be removed — help is available!

TIP

Access the following mental health resources for further help.

Phone:

- Lifeline 13 11 14
- Beyond Blue 1300 22 46 36
- Kids Helpline 1800 55 1800
- Grief Line 1300 845 745

Online:

- www.beyondblue.org.au
- www.blackdoginstitute.org.au/resources-support
- www.reachout.com

Working on your brain health

Have you ever thought how much you rely on your brain for your day-to-day function? Your brain serves as the main control panel for your body and influences all the functions of your vital organs. You need your brain so you can think, reason, remember, learn and communicate. If your brain isn't functioning properly, you know you are in real trouble!

Many experts struggle to define exactly what is meant by 'brain health'. I have even heard one esteemed professor in the United Kingdom describe brain health in an interview as simply having 'a brain that is healthy and free from disease'. While this does seem quite straightforward, it really highlights the difficulty in knowing exactly what we mean by 'keeping your brain healthy'.

In chapter 2, I highlight that dementia (including Alzheimer's disease) is the second most common cause of death for men in Australia. For women, dementia and Alzheimer's disease are, in fact, the number one cause.

Many studies have looked at what contributes to brain health and the decline in cognitive function. While age might be blamed as one of the inevitable causes, undoubtedly a link exists between many of the lifestyle behaviours that contribute to other metabolic diseases, which can then also influence brain health. For example, high blood pressure, obesity, poor nutrition and lack of social connectivity have been associated with the more likely onset of Alzheimer's and dementia. Other poor lifestyle choices such as alcohol consumption, drug use or smoking are also associated with earlier cognitive decline.

In the past, testing for brain health has not been as easy as undergoing other health tests, such as those for heart health, diabetes or bowel cancer. However, some very recent advances look at brain blood supply as well as the retina blood vessels, which can be examined through a detailed eye inspection. This provides a direct pathway to the brain and some promising advances in eye testing have identified early indicators that may predict signs of developing dementia and Alzheimer's disease.

By recognising these changes, you can introduce lifestyle practices such as exercise, better nutrition and weight loss. You can also add cognitive challenges associated with social connectivity and social interaction. For example, playing cards, and completing word puzzles and crosswords challenge the brain and have been shown to help it continue to function in a healthy way. Consider your brain just as you would any other dynamic structure in your body — for example, your muscles. Your brain similarly needs challenges, stimulation and 'workouts' to maintain, grow and improve. Muscles slow down and lose strength as we age. and so does the brain. Regular problem solving, reading, learning a new language, jigsaw puzzles, dancing — the list of brain-health-promoting activities is endless.

'Use it or lose it' is advice that can be applied to many of the body's functions over your lifetime — and the brain is no exception!

So, if you want to keep your brain health optimised, the principles are very similar to those you need to apply to keep the rest of your body in good shape. (See also chapter 7 for some tips on which foods that are beneficial for healthy brain function.)

Alzheimer's update

While scientists still don't really understood why certain individuals develop Alzheimer's disease and dementia symptoms later in life and others are spared, these two conditions remain a major source of disability and death in the community.

Research is actively underway to try to identify better ways of testing for Alzheimer's, but recent reports that new early detection methods are on the way is certainly encouraging. Recent studies have suggested a blood biomarker might help identify individuals who are predisposed to developing Alzheimer's disease later in life. The biomarker for Alzheimer's is known as 3HAA and has been worked on by the research laboratory at Macquarie University in NSW. This research found that people who carried high levels of this biomarker were 35 times more likely to develop Alzheimer's and dementia in the future.

(continued)

I have previously mentioned that many illnesses, such as cardiac disease, have well-established medical checks you can undertake. In the past, mental illness and other brain conditions such as dementia and Alzheimer's have been difficult to detect early. Hopefully, this latest screening development will be verified and become available as an accessible mainstream health check tool. Watch this space!

Protecting your epigenome

What is the epigenome, and how do you protect it?

You've likely heard of the concept of your DNA determining your genetic make-up and contributing to your background health risks. Your DNA is an inherited characteristic from your parents, grandparents and other ancestors, and is considered the core building blocks of your make-up. However, your DNA is also influenced by a substance called the epigenome, which surrounds and shields your DNA, allowing it to be 'preserved' for as long as possible. And your epigenome can be influenced by lifestyle factors such as exercise, diet and stress.

While your DNA is fixed in its structure, the epigenome surrounding and protecting your DNA can change a lot throughout a lifetime and, in fact, health scientists believe the deterioration in the epigenome causes many of the aging changes that we normally associate with advancing years. The secret is to make sure that the epigenome does a great job so that the effects of aging are minimised and slowed down, particularly as you get into the later years of approaching 100 and beyond.

Poor lifestyle choices can mean that the epigenome does not function at its optimal capacity, while good lifestyle choices mean the epigenome does a much better job. In this way, by nurturing the epigenome, you have the ability to control the type of aging processes in your body. The epigenome also plays an important role in switching on and off other genes in the body so that they function at their best. So even though you may not be able to alter your DNA, you can certainly influence your epigenome function and, therefore, have a positive effect on the way your genetic make-up performs during your lifetime and the influence it has on your health predictors.

The concept of epigenetics has been around for many decades, but it has only been in more recent years that ground-breaking research has determined just how much you can control the health of your epigenome and, therefore, our overall body health and wellbeing.

Scientists now know the epigenome can be damaged by many lifestyle behaviours and undergo chemical change. One of the changes that can occur at a chemical level is methylation of the epigenome, causing it to switch off and not function properly. This can increase your risk of several negative consequences, including cancer, kidney disease and blood defects. Methylation of the DNA molecule also results in damage and contributes to the DNA unravelling, which then progresses the aging process. While many chemical processes can damage DNA and the epigenome, it is the methylation process that is attracting most research in the scientific world, as experts work to find how to reverse this process. By protecting the epigenome, you can take one further step on your pathway to a longer healthier life.

Again, the message is simple—lifestyle choices such as poor nutrition, lack of exercise, smoking, and poor environmental conditions including pollution can result in damage to your epigenome and contribute to a combination of physical and mental health disorders. Your immune system can also be damaged through these processes, which then has an impact across a wide range of health conditions. Many of the major pharmaceutical companies in the world are actively working with research agencies to discover medications that can reverse the epigenome methylation and other DNA-damaging processes. This is certainly an exciting area of medical research and will develop further over the coming decade.

Boosting your immunity

Your body requires a high-functioning immune system for its survival. The topic of immunity has been at the forefront of global health discussions ever since the emergence of the COVID-19 pandemic threat in 2020. Your risk of falling ill from any infection threat, viral or otherwise and including COVID-19, depends on the level of resistance your body is able to mount against that infection threat.

The white cells system in your bloodstream primarily provides the immune cells, with the main type of immunity cell known as a 'lymphocyte'. The body has many types of resistance, but the primary immune lymphocyte system utilises B cells, T cells and the scarily named NK ('natural killer') cells.

The more 'tuned up' or 'alert' your lymphocyte immune system is, the lower your risk of succumbing to an infection challenge such as the common cold, influenza, other respiratory infections or common viruses. In other words, the healthier your immune system, the better your body's response to a challenge.

You can boost your body's natural immune system in many ways, and all of these are covered in more detail through this book. Happily, all these measures are also associated with many other health-promoting benefits, which is why they are in my 'Healthy 100' list.

For now, you can use the following key strategies (backed by science) to help boost your immune system to its optimal healthy level:

- exercise (my favourite topic!)

- eat healthily—focus on rainbow foods and increasing antioxidants

- get quality sleep

- avoid smoking

- increase your social connectivity

- practise meditation and relaxation

- get a pet

- laugh

- enjoy healthy, consensual sex

- maintain a positive, optimistic outlook.

A highly functioning immune system keeps you healthier for a greater percentage of the time. Conversely, a poor immune system makes you more prone to the myriad infection risks you can be confronted with over a lifetime. By adopting measures to keep your immune system as healthy as possible, you are taking a further step on your pathway to promoting a longer, healthier and more productive life.

Key takeaways

Most of the conditions discussed in this chapter will be familiar to you. Understanding the common ailments and chronic illnesses helps you avoid them, and take measures in your healthy lifestyle practices to minimise the risks. One of the important measures is having regular health check-ups to identify any predisposing risks. Armed with this knowledge and potential interventions, you can take the necessary steps to help ensure you not only live longer but also remain healthy for as long as possible in your remaining years—the true meaning of healthspan.

4

Health issues for men and women

In recent times, it seems that men's health gets more publicity than the corresponding topic of women's health. Most men certainly do need to have more awareness of their own health and potential health issues — historically, women have tended to take more responsibility for their own health from a younger age and get their required health check-ups, usually from the onset of puberty. This has not been the case with men.

Men typically do not think about their health maintenance early enough. Just because you never think about your health, however, doesn't mean you will stay healthy forever. In this case, ignorance is not bliss!

Illness does not discriminate among genders and while some specific conditions may occur more in men than women, and others more in women than in men, a huge range of common conditions also need to be checked for in both genders. Men need to understand that they can have more influence over their health than they realise by taking a positive attitude to health promotion. The adage that 'prevention is better (and cheaper) than cure' applies to men and women — and to so many of the health conditions I discuss in this book. In addition, preventive strategies are generally more pleasant than the available treatment options if you need intervention for a condition detected later than it should be.

Men still aren't living as long as women

Here's a startling statement: men and women are different! This is not likely to be news to you, and you may also be aware that women, in general, outlive men. The topic has been the subject of many jokes over the years, and I expect you are familiar with many of them. I will spare you the humour and concentrate on what is known. Unfortunately, the different lifespans of men and women is still a somewhat complex question in the scientific world.

According to the latest data from the Australian Bureau of Statistics (ABS) and Australian Institute of Health and Welfare (AIHW), a female born in 2021 has a life expectancy of 85.3 years. A male has a life expectancy of 81.2 years — a difference of 4.1 years. Compare this with 50 years ago when the female 'advantage' was 6.3 years. The gap is closing, but it is certainly happening slowly. But what are the reasons for the difference?

The simple answer is that it is a multifactorial explanation, but the three primary contributors are as follows:

1. *Hormonal factors:* This theory is based on the oestrogen effect in women, especially in the pre-menopausal phases of life.

Oestrogen levels are much higher in women than in men, and this is associated with a lower lipid profile and a more likely increase in good cholesterol (HDL). In addition, oestrogen has a direct effect on blood vessel health, which in turn affects important areas such as heart health, brain health, diabetes and renal function. Cardiac death remains a leading cause of death in both men and women, but certainly men are at higher risk (although the gap is narrowing globally).

2. *Genetic reasons:* The role of genetics has been postulated in relation to improved female lifespan and healthspan. The **XX** female chromosome combination is more stable, whereas the **XY** male chromosome combination results in some denaturing and instability of the Y chromosome as men age. Studies of telomere health show that females have longer telomeres, which help to stabilise their DNA and leads to reduced age-related cellular changes. (Refer to chapter 1 for more on telomeres and aging.) The shrinking of the male Y chromosome with advancing years causes higher aging risks in the male population.

3. *Behaviour and environmental factors:* Again, this is a complex issue, but on a global scale, men have increased incidence of smoking, alcohol consumption and risk-taking behaviour. Males engaged in certain occupations also have increased exposure to dangerous carcinogens. Furthermore, women are more likely to seek interventions for illness much earlier than men. This allows them to achieve earlier detection, meaning more effective treatment programs can begin at an earlier point in the illness. This earlier intervention results in better outcomes and reduced risk of death.

While these factors have been linked with increased female survival in the specific conditions just mentioned, these benefits likely also apply across a range of other illness conditions and hence provide an overall advantage to women. Poor lifestyle choices can certainly negate some of the effects, but the hormonal and chromosomal components are undoubtedly a contributing factor to lifespan expectations.

Most men certainly do need to have more awareness of their own health and potential health issues — as mentioned, women have tended to take more responsibility for their own health. I believe this is a result of women being more 'tuned in' to their body's function and the health checks required from a younger age than men. From the onset of puberty, women are better educated on the need for regular health check-ups, particularly in the reproductive health areas such as cervical, ovarian and breast health. As a result of being more informed about seeking these check-ups, the likelihood of detecting problems at a younger age increases due to the more frequent contact women have with their health adviser. This more frequent contact also increases the likelihood of other health issues being detected.

Of course, in more recent times the stereotypical 'male breadwinner' role is not as common, and women are now frequently the primary income earner in many households. Overall, women's role in paid work has increased — and so too has the dilemma for some of balancing home, motherhood, perhaps caring for elderly parents and pursuing their career. This has added to the challenge for women of looking after their personal health.

Why men avoid health check-ups

Men avoiding health check-ups is generally a global trend. However, when looking at the reasons behind this, we do have some 'Aussie' quirks. We live in a somewhat 'macho' male culture in Australia, where men would traditionally rather 'suck it up' and put up with persistent minor—or even moderate—symptoms before seeking medical advice. Many people feel uncomfortable seeking medical advice about something they consider to be 'just a niggle', or not that serious. This is even more so the case for Australian men, and especially older Australian men, who often leave seeking this advice too late, so their treatment options become more limited, more expensive and, often, more unpleasant.

Men will also use the excuse of the pressure of working life and the need to be in a traditional 'breadwinner' role, arguing this prevents them from having the time to visit their family practitioner during standard business hours. They may also adopt the attitude of a false sense of illness immunity, believing that 'it won't happen to me'. The old approach of, 'If it ain't broke, don't service it' is not the attitude to be taken when it comes to personal body maintenance. I suspect a fear of the unknown also exists among many men that prevents them from seeking advice as readily as women do.

This traditional reluctance needs to change. Why? The simple fact is that many men were (and still are) dying due to a lack of awareness of medical conditions that could have been detected with a proper health assessment. We are now much more aware of the benefits of early detection in preventing death. We know we can offset much of the pain and anxiety of illness through early treatment of many of the conditions that traditionally caused death in our parents or grandparents. In addition, we've seen many advances in the treatments available once a condition has been detected.

The bottom line is that men need to take a more positive attitude to health prevention. It is a positive investment—not only for their own health, but also for their family, loved ones, business and other dependents in their life.

Men's health and ASOSS

I have observed various 'behaviour cycles' related to men's health over many years, with each cycle being the focus of various health education campaigns. I have summarised these into five stages, represented by the acronym ASOSS:

+ *Alcohol:* While alcohol excess is an ongoing issue still in today's society, certainly in the 1960s and 1970s it was a major concern, particularly for men, with conditions such as liver cirrhosis, alcoholic brain damage and domestic violence being linked with alcohol use in the community.

+ *Smoking:* In the 1980s the health education focus became one of publicising the health risks of smoking. Ironically, doctors were used to actively promote and even advertise smoking in the 1960s and 1970s, but the research on its harmful effects is unchallenged now and the health risks well accepted.

+ *Obesity:* The health education emphasis in recent years has moved from anti-smoking campaigns to the risks of obesity and highlighting the links the condition has to multiple illnesses — for example, heart disease, diabetes and cancers. Obesity is also a risk for women, with rates of women overweight or obese catching up with those of men.

+ *Sedentary:* Lifestyle changes and technological advances over the last 30 years have resulted in people being much less physically active. The number of people in sedentary occupations has increased, as has the proportion of the population seeking passive recreation entertainment options. According to 2018 data from the Australian Bureau of Statistics, this has meant the proportion of community members — men and women — who are not participating in sufficient regular physical activity has risen to 55 per cent. For those over 65 years of age, the figure is a staggering 73 per cent. Research shows physical activity is one of the most important interventions in health promotion and contributes to prevention of many of the current causes of illness and death in society.

+ *Sugar:* While blood lipids (including cholesterol) have been a focus of nutritional education for many years, the more recent emphasis has been on excessive sugar in the diet and the negative impact this can have on risk factors for ill health. Excess sugar intake (in the form of glucose, sucrose and fructose, and often hidden in many foods) has been liked to chronic medical conditions such as obesity, heart disease and diabetes. Again, these risks apply equally to men and women.

However, one condition — which I believe is a major contributor to community and particularly men's health behaviour not improving — does not receive much publicity.

I have termed this condition 'LRD', which stands for 'listener receptor deficit'! This condition simply refers to the fact that many people (but again particularly men) do not listen to the advice given to them! My concern is the failure of people to act upon the information being provided to them in relation to personal health. Simply put, every person needs to step up and take responsibility for improving their health. Don't ignore the scientifically established habits (outlined throughout this book) that promote healthy longevity!

Focusing in on prostate disease

When the topic of 'men's health' is mentioned, one of the first conditions that most people think of is prostate health and the concern about prostate cancer. Sometimes I think men think of the prostate more commonly than they do heart disease when considering their personal health. Of course, their concern is warranted, and the need for men to regularly check for prostate health and undergo screening is paramount.

In 2021 prostate cancer rated as the third most common cause of cancer death in Australia (after lung and bowel cancer). The AIHW estimated the number of new cases diagnosed in 2021 was 18 110. This represents 23 per cent of all new male cancer cases diagnosed. The number of estimated deaths in 2021 was 3323 males, representing 12 per cent of all male cancer deaths.

The Australian Cancer Council estimates that a male has a one in eight (13 per cent) risk of being diagnosed with prostate cancer by the age of 85. The number of men currently living with prostate cancer in Australia is estimated to be around 89 000, due to diagnoses made in the past five years.

Fortunately, deaths from prostate cancer are declining as detection and screening processes become more utilised — meaning the cancer is diagnosed at an earlier stage, making survival more likely. With advancements in treatment and early detection of prostate disease, the chance of surviving at least five years after diagnosis has been gradually increasing — from around 61 per cent in 1988 to around 96 per cent in 2021.

The message for men is clear — you should begin screening for prostate cancer early, possibly from as early as 35 years of age, particularly if you have a family history of prostate cancer. The earlier the diagnosis, the better your chance of an excellent prognosis and long-term survival.

Screening for prostate disease begins with a simple discussion with your GP around any known family history and the common symptoms of prostate dysfunction, which include frequent urination or poor urinary stream. Your doctor may conduct a DRE (digital rectal examination), which checks for the size and texture of the prostate. You may also be offered a prostate blood test, known as a 'PSA' (prostate-specific antigen). This has been available for many decades but was introduced in the early 1990s as a method of widespread screening. (The test was a major factor in the dramatic increase in the early detection of prostate cancer and the significant positive reduction in the incidence of fatal disease including metastatic prostate cancer.) In more recent times, MRI scanning and PET scanning have been introduced to look at the prostate gland morphology and detect abnormal prostate areas.

It is recommended that PSA blood screening begins at least at age 40, particularly if you have a positive family history. All men over 50 years should be tested regularly.

Several strategies are also available to reduce the risk of developing prostate cancer. People who regularly exercise and are non-smokers have a much lower incidence of prostate cancer. A healthy diet, including avoidance of heavily processed and high carbohydrate foods, is also important. So concentrate on eating healthy fats and increasing your consumption of unprocessed foods including vegetables and fruits. Even the consumption of regular caffeine has been linked to having positive benefits for prostate cancer health.

One thing you might find pleasing is the revelation from multiple studies that males who experience a higher number of ejaculations in their lifetime have a much lower incidence of prostate cancer. Absolutely true! This certainly appears to be welcome news for most men!

The bottom line?

Make sure you have regular health check-ups, including a prostate check. Survival rates are much higher, and the incidence of death from prostate cancer dramatically reduced with this strategy — meaning you have one more solution in the puzzle of extending your healthspan to 100 years and beyond.

Health issues for women

As noted, women tend to see their GP more regularly and be more aware of potential health issues, but checks can still slip through. Women (like men) can also delay seeking advice because they feel a new symptom or health change is not serious enough to raise with their doctor. Women can get caught up in their busy lives just as easily as men — and regular screenings can slip through and routine blood tests might not be followed up on. And, especially as they age and enter perimenopause — while continuing to care for children and perhaps elderly parents — women may start to wonder whether feeling tired and rundown is just their new norm.

Through all of these changes, women need to continue to take charge of their health, and speak to their GP about anything that's worrying them — even the small 'niggles' and concerns.

Here's a run through of some specific health issues for women:

- *Breast cancer:* As mentioned in chapter 3, 2022 saw 20 640 new cases of breast cancer in Australia, and the vast majority of these cases were in women. BreastScreen Australia, a joint initiative of the Australian and state and territory governments, offers women over 40 a free mammogram every two years. They actively invite women aged 50 to 74 to screen. For more information on this program and to find a BreastScreen location near you, go to www.health.gov.au/our-work/breastscreen-australia-program.

- *Cervical cancer:* New cases of cervical cancer are much lower than those of breast cancer, with the AIHW estimating 2022 saw 942 new cases of cervical cancer diagnosed in Australia. In part, this low number is due to improved screening approaches. The new, more accurate, cervical screening test was introduced in Australia in 2017, replacing the Pap test. This test only needs to be performed every five years, with the Australian government recommending it for all women aged between 25 and 75.

- *Reproductive health:* This is a very broad area covering contraception options, painful and/or irregular periods, and health care before, during and following pregnancy. Your GP is your first port of call for any questions or concerns in this area, including issues such as endometriosis, uterine fibroids and taking longer than 12 months to conceive when trying to become pregnant.

- *Iron and ferritin levels:* Iron is needed in the body to make haemoglobin, a protein in red blood cells that carries oxygen from the lungs to all parts of the body, and myoglobin, a protein that provides oxygen to muscles. Ferritin levels reflect the iron stores available in the body. Women who have just given birth, follow a plant-based diet and/or have heavy or prolonged periods are at risk of having low iron and ferritin levels — and so feeling tired and rundown all the time. Female athletes can also be at high risk of poor nutrition habits, which includes low iron intake especially if they avoid the best source of dietary iron—lean red meat. Your GP can order a blood test to check your iron and ferritin levels, and can advise on possible strategies based on your results.

- *Hormonal changes leading up to menopause:* The time before a woman's periods stop completely is known as perimenopause—and it can last for up to 10 years. (The average length of perimenopause is four to six years.) A common feature of perimenopause is irregular periods, but other symptoms include hot flushes, mood swings, low libido, sore breasts, weight gain and vaginal dryness. Again, your GP is the best person to talk to about any of these symptoms. They will be able to advise on lifestyle changes that may help—including, you guessed it, eating a healthy diet, doing regular exercise and getting enough sleep. Common themes throughout this book! Your GP can also advise on contraception during perimenopause and chat with you about potential hormone replacement therapy (HRT). HRT is used to restore levels of the hormones oestrogen and progesterone, and improve symptoms and quality of life, but must be considered in the context of a woman's overall health status and whether other potential risks are present—for example, a family history of breast cancer.

- *Osteoporosis:* This condition causes bones to become thin, weak and fragile, and it is more common in women than men—according to the AIHW, 29 per cent of women aged 75 and over have the condition versus 10 per cent of men. It's also a condition that is under-diagnosed, due to it not having overt symptoms. However, the AIHW reports that osteoporosis was recorded as an underlying or associated cause for 2366 deaths in Australia in 2021, representing 1.4 per cent of all deaths and 26 per cent of all musculoskeletal deaths. The condition can be diagnosed with a simple bone density scan (known as a DEXA scan). After diagnosis, your GP can advise on possible treatment options, including lifestyle changes, controlled exercise (including resistance training), increasing calcium and vitamin D, and medication.

TIP

Some studies have shown that hormone replacement therapy, used to reduce symptoms of perimenopause and improve quality of life, can lead to a slightly increased risk of developing breast cancer. However, other studies have suggested that specific options can *lower* your risk of breast cancer. These risks are also influenced by specific health factors, and this is why it's best to have a full discussion with your GP before making any decisions.

Women and physical appearance pressures

While men are also starting to be more concerned about their looks and body shape, women are still more likely to feel the pressure of societal physical appearance demands, often inappropriately promoted by social media 'influencers'. Following fad diets and poor nutritional practices in an effort to become thinner only add to the stress on many women.

In my work as a specialist sport and exercise physician, I have often worked with female sporting individuals and teams. The incidence of eating disorders and body image issues can be very high, particularly in certain high-demand activities such as gymnastics, ballet and distance running. While these

(continued)

challenges are not exclusive to women, the number of people affected by unhealthy practices is higher among females.

Issues of low bone density, iron deficiency and hormonal disturbances are all well documented in women with poor nutrition practices, regardless of whether they are engaged in sport or not. Their long-term health often suffers physically and emotionally, including poor self-esteem. No magic potion, pill or single workout machine can provide women (or men for that matter) with the perfect, slim body as seen in so many fashion and lifestyle magazines or online posts. Don't beat up on yourself—be the best 'you' you can be, through healthy lifestyle practices that are achievable and, more importantly, sustainable for your situation.

Mental health issues for men and women

Recently, the standard health check-up has been expanded to also include assessments for emotional and spiritual health, due the large impact that mental illness has had on society and people's ability to function at an optimal level. Indeed, I've never known a time in my medical career when the focus on mental health has been as strong as it has been in the last 10 years. The incidence of mental and emotional health issues in society is also better documented.

According to the National Study of Mental Health and Wellbeing 2020–22 (released by the Australian Bureau of Statistics in October 2023):

- 17.4 per cent of Australians (3.4 million people) aged 16 to 85 years saw a health professional for mental health concerns in the past 12 months.

- One in four women (24.6 per cent) had a 12-month mental disorder in 2020–2022, compared with almost one in five men (18.3 per cent).

- Females experienced higher rates than males of anxiety disorders (21.1 per cent compared with 13.3 per cent) and affective disorders (8.6 per cent compared with 6.5 per cent).

- Males had over twice the rate of substance use disorders (4.4 per cent compared with 2.1 per cent).

- More females (21.6 per cent) than males (12.9 per cent) saw a health professional for mental health concerns.

However, incidences of mental health issues are still under reported. Many people are still reluctant to seek help or get advice when they're struggling. This needs to change!

Traditionally, women have been better equipped at communicating problems, and so have been more likely to open up and share their concerns with friends and colleagues compared to men. Conversely, the traditional macho image that men may feel pushed to live up to has been one of maintaining a stoic attitude. This often meant men were more likely to suppress any emotional difficulties — often with tragic ultimate outcomes.

Males are still three times more likely to take their own life than females. In 2022, the AIHW reported 2455 male deaths from suicide, at a rate of 18.8 per 100 000; the same year saw 794 female deaths at a rate of 5.9 per 100 000. In 2022, the number of deaths by suicide was higher for males than females in all reported age groups. Alarmingly, suicide remains the leading cause of death for Australians aged 15 to 44.

For men and women alike, lifting the stigma of seeking assistance when it is required is an important goal. Indeed, one of the great advances in recent years has been the number of services and organisations available for people to discuss their problems. It just takes the first brave step to seek them out, and you can find some possible options in the nearby breakout box.

All levels of government (state and federal) have acknowledged the need to assist with funding support services. Conditions such as depression, anxiety, insomnia and burnout are common to both men and women, and anyone who is struggling deserves to get the professional medical assistance they need.

TIP

If you know or recognise someone who you think needs help, reach out to them for a chat. Start with an 'are you okay?' question, but also dig another layer deeper. Ask them, 'How is work?', 'How's the home life?', 'Are you feeling up to your best?' You may be surprised at the honest answers you get back.

Mental health resources

If you're struggling with your mental or emotional health, telephone or online mental health resources can often be effective, especially if you aren't able to access a health service, or find talking to someone face to face difficult. Here are some telephone and online resources to try:

+ Lifeline is for anyone having a personal crisis — call 13 11 14 or chat online at www.lifeline.org.au

+ MensLine Australia is an online counselling and forum option for men — call 1300 78 99 78 or go to www.mensline.org.au

+ Dads In Distress offers peer support for separated dads — call 1300 853 437 or check out www.parentsbeyondbreakup.com/dids

+ Head to Health is a federal government service that can connect you to local mental health services — call 1800 595 212 or go to www.headtohealth.gov.au

+ SANE Australia is for people living with a mental illness, and their families — call 1800 187 263 or chat online at www.sane.org

+ Beyond Blue offers many health resources, including those designed specifically for teens, parents and men — call 1300 22 4636 or chat online at www.beyondblue.org.au

+ Moodgym is a free online cognitive behaviour therapy program to help you manage symptoms of depression and anxiety — go to www.moodgym.com.au

+ If you are experiencing mental health issues related to your sexuality or gender identity, Qlife provides a counselling and referral service for LGBTIQA+ people — go to www.lgbtiqhealth.org.au/qlife

Key takeaways

The key components of good health for men are regular exercise, healthy nutrition, social connectivity, personal development and avoidance of high-risk-taking behaviours such as smoking. Regular health check-ups, including screening for any heart or prostate issues, are a must. Opening up about mental and emotional health issues—and seeking help if needed—is also important.

While women tend to be better at monitoring their health, important check-ups can still be delayed and worries ignored. Regular exercise, healthy nutrition and social connectivity are equally important for women, and they need to continue to be aware of when they should be seeing their GP and what new treatments may be available during different stages of life—such as perimenopause.

I cover regular check-ups in the following chapter, and the whole of part III offers valuable tips on improving your exercise, nutrition and social connectivity.

5

Checking your health — the why, how and when

I am always pleased when a patient takes the initiative and enquires about obtaining a 'complete health check-up'. While the actual components of this might vary depending on individual circumstances, some key issues need to be addressed. The extent and range of testing undertaken can then be tailored depending on the individual's health status and specific needs.

In principle, the concept of a health check-up is to detect any risk factors or early warning signs of illness, which can then result in early intervention to avoid progression of the problem. When detected early, many medical conditions — including heart disease, cancer and diabetes — can be treated at least in part by lifestyle modifications, which can lead to a significant minimisation of the risk of the disease progressing. These modifications may include weight loss, nutrition changes and the introduction of an exercise program. Some lifestyle modifications may even reverse the risk of complications — for example, when dealing with conditions such as high blood pressure, borderline diabetes problems and cholesterol issues. Certain medications may still be needed to correct an abnormality discovered during testing, but often the need for higher doses of traditional medications can be offset with these lifestyle modifications.

In chapter 1, I outline the top 10 causes of death for men and women in Australia. These include coronary artery disease, dementia, stroke, and lung, prostate, breast and bowel cancer. While testing for every potential medical condition may not be justified, it is important to identify the most common causes of illness and mortality in the community and test for these — and then implement lifestyle changes and care as needed.

In this chapter, I run through what you can expect from a health check-up, how often you might need to see your doctor, and how you can start to put some preventative measures in place to reduce the need for your doctor to prescribe new medicines at each check-up.

Understanding what a health check entails

The complexity of the health check required depends on your medical background and your age. As a rule, if you're still under 40, you do not require sophisticated check-ups unless you have a strong family history of particular medical conditions. After age 40 your family medical practitioner/GP can conduct a simple questionnaire on your background health and lifestyle, along with a basic office examination. From there, your doctor can determine if any early indications or risk factors are present for common serious illnesses such as heart disease, stroke, cancers and diabetes, and if any special tests are required — for example, cardiac screening or bowel colonoscopy. A mental health assessment should also be a critical part of this assessment.

The components of a 'proper' health check include:

1. *An honest and open chat:* Your GP will ask you about your past and current health, family history and lifestyle, and chat with you about your mental and emotional health. Specific questions will focus on past medical illnesses, smoking, nutrition practices, exercise patterns, sleep and emotional health.

2. *A basic office physical examination:* While this can be limited in its scope, it will generally include a blood pressure check, pulse rate and rhythm, heart sounds, abdominal exam (liver, spleen, kidney and other masses) and basic skin exam. Height, weight, BMI (body mass index) and waist circumference are still used to establish baseline information, despite some limitations in their accuracy. A simple urine check can be used to assess for the presence of blood or protein in the urine, and help assess kidney function,

3. *Blood tests:* These would initially look at the following:
   - full blood examination — including haemoglobin, white cells, haematocrit — often referred to as 'blood count'
   - liver function
   - renal (kidney) function
   - lipid profile — fasting (including good HDL and bad LDL cholesterol levels)
   - blood glucose level — fasting

- prostate-specific antigen (PSA) — males only
- insulin levels
- iron profile — particularly if experiencing heavy periods, fatigue, following a strict non-meat diet or in pregnancy
- inflammatory markers — more likely if concerns exist about an autoimmune inflammatory disorder or disease
- other blood markers depending on the individual's health status.

4. *Specific tests:* Your doctor will determine if any more standard screening tests are needed, based on your risk profile and time since previous screening. These may include:
   - chest X-ray
   - heart CTA (computerised tomography angiogram; a type of imaging angiogram) and cardiac calcium score to look at plaque deposit in the important coronary arteries
   - colonoscopy to check for bowel polyps, cancer
   - detailed skin check with dermatologist
   - breast exam
   - testicular exam
   - cervical screening for cervical cancer (women only — this can be performed by your GP)
   - other tests, such as abdominal or breast ultrasound, mammogram or CT scan if a lump or mass is detected.

For a targeted cardiac health check, a detailed history and office examination should be performed. Depending on clinical indications, other cardiac screening tests may also be needed, such as the heart CTA and calcium score included in the preceding list. An exercise echocardiogram may also be used, which is a functional test observing the heart perform under some exercise load — for example, on a treadmill or exercise bike. More detailed angiogram studies could be undertaken if specific cardiac symptoms are suggestive of more serious coronary artery narrowing.

Your doctor will determine which of these specific tests are needed once they've assessed your health profile.

Timing your check-ups

The exact age you should start booking in for these check-ups is debatable, but in my mind it is never too early to get some basic information about your future health risk factors.

In practice, if you are between 20 and 30 years old, you do not need any complex medical check-ups but should at least develop a relationship with a trusted family doctor. This will allow you to seek out information on matters such as vaccinations and contraception, and manage all the common simple illnesses such as respiratory or gastric infections that you may experience in everyday life. Women will need to book in for regular cervical screening (every five years) and breast exams.

Between the ages of 30 and 40 years, testing becomes more important and you may need to look at specific assessments, particularly if you have a positive family history of any of the common disorders such as breast cancer or bowel cancer. Most health practitioners would agree that over the age of 40 a regular health check becomes more important and recommended.

If you're currently inactive, in sedentary work or have any known medical conditions, also book in for a health check before starting any exercise — again, especially if you're over 40. Your doctor will run through the kinds of checks outlined in the previous section, and also chat with you about the level and intensity of exercise you're safe to start out doing. Any specific restrictions can be identified to assist in selecting the appropriate type and intensity of your initial workouts. They can also help you track your strength and fitness gains as you progress, and give you the go ahead to move on to more intense exercise options. (See the following chapter for more on a medical screening before commencing exercise.)

The frequency at which you have these tests would also be determined by your age and the initial results. If everything is normal, for example, your doctor may request you get checked again in two years. If an issue pops up, you may need check-ups every year or even more regularly.

When any adverse findings are only slightly outside the accepted range, simple lifestyle interventions such as weight loss, dietary changes and exercise can have dramatic improvements on returning the abnormality to normal levels. On occasions medications may be required for significant abnormalities, but these need to be discussed with your family doctor.

Building your own pharmacy

You likely don't realise you have a very comprehensive pharmacy under your own roof. It is your own body!

When you think of purchasing medical supplies from a pharmacy, your thoughts might typically turn to medications to treat pain, blood pressure, heart disease, high cholesterol (lipids), diabetes, upper respiratory infections — the list goes on. If we look at the annual cost of medicines purchased in Australia, including government subsidised prescriptions, the cost amounts to billions of dollars. According to the

Australian Institute of Health and Welfare (AIHW), in 2020–21, the Australian federal government recorded $13.9 billion in spending on all subsidised **PBS** and **RPBS** medicines (with **PBS** accounting for 98 per cent of the total), or $541 per person. Consumers then paid an additional $3.2 billion towards their **PBS** and **RPBS** prescriptions (for both above and under co-payment prescriptions).

Of these medicines, those used to treat cardiovascular conditions were the most commonly dispensed (33 per cent of all **PBS** and **RPBS** prescriptions), with a government spend of $1.1 billion for 2020–21. The next most common medicines prescribed were those used to treat nervous and mental health disorders (23 per cent of prescriptions), with a government spend of $1.3 billion for 2020–21.

These everyday medical compounds have a common mechanism of action. They are chemicals directed at re-establishing, balancing or lowering abnormal levels of dysfunctional hormones in the body. Individuals vary dramatically in their response to these medications and it is often a challenge to get the dose right before seeing any positive benefit in correcting an abnormal health finding.

Throughout this book, I outline how your body is capable of making natural hormones and chemicals that replicate the benefits of these synthetic pharmaceutical medicines. My pet topic of physical activity and exercise again comes to the fore here. Improvements to the metabolic processes seen from regular exercise are often brought about through the regulation and production of the body's own natural health hormones (true 'organic' medicines).

Conditions such as high blood pressure, high cholesterol, high blood sugar, depression, anxiety and sleep disturbance can all be positively influenced by a regular exercise program. Exercise produces chemicals, including neurotransmitters (e.g. dopamine), which have a similar action to the artificially produced pharmaceutical products — and it is much cheaper to obtain these through a regular exercise program than it is by spending money at your local pharmacy.

Let me make it perfectly clear: I am not suggesting that people with a significant health condition should go against medical advice and not use the medications prescribed under the care of their family doctor or specialist. However, by combining these medications with a regular exercise program, many people have been shown to get an enhanced response to their medication and in some cases to be able to reduce the required dose of their medication. Improvements in blood pressure levels, blood sugar control and reductions in unhealthy lipid profiles are all positive outcomes from regular exercise and may help you minimise the need for additional medical supplementation through your doctor's prescription. These benefits accrue as your fitness level improves with consistent exercise activity.

It is important to speak with your doctor if you are on regular medications for any health disorder. Ask your doctor about the additional role exercise could play in assisting with managing your condition as well as helping to keep any medications at the minimum effective amount required.

> ## TIP
> Your body is your best pharmacy — it produces 'natural medicines' so you can have control over your own health.

A regular exercise program provides more benefits than the simple goals of weight loss or changing muscle tone. These additional benefits of exercise are extraordinary and well documented, and I outline them in more detail in chapter 6.

So next time you are heading to your medicine cabinet to reach for some medication, take a look in the mirror that is hopefully attached to that cupboard, and you will see that one of the most important medical 'suppliers' is staring straight back at you. Take control!

Key takeaways

My take home message is simple: the sooner you become aware of a medical problem, the sooner you can seek advice on treating it. Regular health check-ups, including screening for any heart, diabetes, breast, cervical or prostate issues, allow this to occur. The solution may be a simple lifestyle adjustment, such as more exercise (my favourite adjustment!) and a realistic weight loss target. Alternatively, further testing can allow your doctor to decide if other measures such as medication are required.

Never underestimate how capable your body is. Treat it well and it will continue to keep you healthy and active right through to the target I have for you all — 100 years and beyond.

PART III

100 ways to improve your healthspan

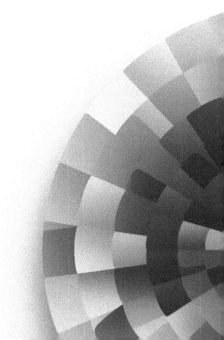

In the chapters in this part, I walk you through 100 ways to improve your lifestyle practices. Remember—your goal is a healthier you, leading to a more productive and happier life, for many more years than the accepted current lifespan predictions. The actions provided here can help you slow the aging process, and keep you youthful for longer—well into your later years. That's what healthspan is all about. A healthy 100 and beyond is the goal!

You don't need to do it all, especially not all at once! What I mean by this is that you don't have to adopt each lifestyle change perfectly, or follow every single tip in the following chapters to achieve a healthy living outcome.

You can pick and choose any number of lifestyle practices to get started, and always come back and adopt more once you're on your way. Hopefully, over the next weeks and months you will adopt many of the tips and health messages delivered in these chapters.

You don't have to be perfect, but the changes outlined here can help improve your current situation. Consider the 100 ways a bit of a buffet of health choices—except you don't need to ration yourself with the options. Look over the healthy choices and decide which ones you can add to your life. You do not have to fill your plate, but the more choices you make, the more likely it is you will add benefit to your lifestyle and health.

6
Exercise

Why am I such a devoted advocate for exercise and physical activity for all individuals regardless of age?

It's quite simple really. As the Greek physician Hippocrates argued back in the 5th century BCE, 'Eating alone will not keep a man well; he must also take exercise. For food and exercise, while possessing opposite qualities, yet work together to produce health.' Exercise is the ultimate health supplement. The scientific evidence showing the health benefits of regular physical exercise are now indisputably proven. Those individuals who are regularly active lead a more healthy and productive life.

Exercise—the most important medicine you can take

What is perhaps most disappointing, but not surprising, is that the evidence supporting the role of exercise and physical activity in contributing to a healthy lifestyle has been available for many decades. It is an unfortunate yet common trait of human nature that, despite this information being regularly publicised and despite people being aware of its availability, the majority of people do not act upon the information. You may even remember 'Norm', the highly publicised cartoon character from the Victorian government's 'Life. Be in it' campaign launched in 1975. Norm was a middle-aged, lethargic, beer-bellied, unfit male. He was a stereotypical caricature and I presume he was considered to be representative of the typical male at that time.

The idea behind the campaign was to motivate everyone, not just fat males, to become more active and improve their health. It was catchy and well presented. The program was considered such a success by the government media spin doctors that it was rolled out nationally by the federal government in 1978, and ran until 1981. Its impact by way of uptake and behaviour change, however, was questionable. One survey of 3960 Australians claimed that 40 per cent had 'thought about becoming more active' after viewing the ads. I would argue that 'thinking' does not always translate to action! A scientific term has even been coined for this disconnect — it is known as the 'intention–behaviour gap'.

The subsequent statistics support me. Community obesity rates have continued to increase since the early 1980s, and both fitness levels and participation in regular physical activity have declined since that time. Even at a global level over the past 20 years, we can see a concerning stability or, in many countries, decline in the percentage of individuals who are inactive or fail to meet even minimum guidelines for basic physical activity. We are failing as a nation (and globally) to take action to improve our health.

As a community we have been, and remain, a predominantly sedentary population. Something must change. What will you do to improve yourself? The rest of this chapter provides plenty of ideas.

EXERCISE

#1
....
Learn how exercise works to improve health

Many components contribute to the reason regular physical activity results in a reduction in illness risk and the promotion of good health. I outline some of these components in the following sections.

Increased basal metabolic rate

During physical activity, your metabolic rate rises. This is associated with increases in heart rate, energy usage, oxygen transfer and muscle activity. What is important to understand is that people who are regularly physically active on a majority of days each week have a higher resting metabolic rate (or basal metabolic rate — BMR) compared to those individuals who are not as active.

In other words, during the time that you are not physically active, you are still burning more calories through increased overall muscle activity and are 'up-regulating' your metabolic rate. You are getting health benefits from the consistent exercise sessions even after they are completed. However, this phenomenon has only been documented in those individuals who exercise on consistent, multiple days each week (ideally four to five), not just occasionally.

Fuel consumption

Exercise requires fuel, particularly for working muscles. Muscles prefer blood glucose for energy but will also use circulating and stored fats. Hence, those calories consumed through healthy nutrition practices will be 'burnt up' during exercise, and this assists with weight control and promotes lean body mass (through a reduction in unhealthy stored body fat).

Muscle tone and strength increase

The inclusion of some regular strength training has a positive benefit on muscle tone and muscle shape, and improves stability, balance and support around joints. This is particularly important in the elderly, but any individual can benefit. In addition, more recent scientific studies have shown that strength training has a positive benefit on heart disease, diabetes, bone health and several cancer types, and provides great mental health benefits.

This is an important discovery and emphasises why you need to have a well-rounded and structured exercise program as part of your weekly routine. Strength training is not simply about changing muscles. See later in this chapter for more information on the value of strength training for overall health.

Biochemical changes

Studies have shown for a long time that exercise can provide a benefit in producing certain 'feel-good' chemicals in the body, including brain chemicals. Endorphins are an opiate-like hormone produced during exercise, and they can give a sense of wellbeing to many individuals. In addition, brain neurotransmitters such as dopamine and serotonin are enhanced by exercise. Because of this, exercise has been shown to be effective with management of mental health disorders as well as improving cognitive performance and memory.

Increased antioxidant production is another benefit of regular exercise and may be linked to the anti-aging effects of exercise as well as contributing to stabilising cell metabolism and cell repair. This may be a critical component in reducing the incidence, severity and spread of cancer processes.

More to come...

Further studies are underway that I am sure will uncover other factors associated with the reasons regular exercise contributes to positive health benefits. Stay tuned!

#2 Use exercise as the ultimate health supplement

Exercise has been shown to have a positive influence on many of the ill health predictors that are known in modern society. As US Air Force Colonel and founder of the Cooper Aerobic Center Dr Kenneth Cooper argued, 'You don't stop exercising because you grow old. You grow old because you stop exercising.' The medical evidence is now verified (led in part by Cooper's own Aerobics Center Longitudinal Studies), not just 'doctor spin'.

Exercise is suitable for all ages and is not expensive (and often is free!). To begin a simple walking program, you only need a comfortable pair of sports shoes and standard comfortable clothing that you no doubt already have in your wardrobe. You do not need an expensive membership to a gymnasium, health club or swimming centre, or expensive equipment such as a carbon fibre bike. Each of these additional 'add-ons' can be beneficial as you get more enthusiastic, but starting out does not need to be an expensive process.

In Australia, exercise is not a Pharmaceutical Benefits Scheme (PBS) item. In other words, it does not come with a government subsidised prescription that you take along to the pharmacy. It does not come in a package or bottle. However, it is something you can practise every day, depending on your goals.

The correct dose of exercise is free from side effects, unlike many other medications prescribed to treat ill health. If you get some advice and a medical check if needed, and start out slowly with the correct amount and intensity, you're unlikely to have any problems.

Exercise can be taken long-term as a health 'supplement' without interruption.

Exercise promotes quality of life and healthy longevity. To get these long-term benefits, you only have to build up to 30 minutes of physical activity using large muscle groups doing a range of different activities on five or more days per week. This represents only 1.5 per cent of your entire weekly time available to you. That's a very small amount to invest in improving your future health destiny.

Finally, exercise is non-seasonal and capable of being full of variety so that you can mix up the type of activities to give you more enjoyment.

What other supplement can give you these incredible benefits?!

#3   Work out if you need medical screening

I am frequently asked about which individuals require a medical screening exam before commencing an exercise program. This is a very valid question, and the answer is that it really depends on your current state of fitness and health.

A number of important considerations need to be looked at to determine whether you need screening and how thorough that screening needs to be. These considerations include:

- *Known medical problems:* If you have known conditions, such as cardiac problems, high blood pressure or diabetes, you need

EXERCISE

to discuss the impact of these conditions with your medical practitioner to determine the type of exercise you need to undertake. All the problems just mentioned can benefit from a gradual, guided exercise program and, in fact, on many occasions the medications traditionally prescribed for them can be reduced to a smaller dose as you develop your own health and fitness program.

- *Medication use:* Certain prescription medications, such as blood thinners and beta blockers (which slow the heart rate), can affect your exercise capacity. Discuss these with your family doctor or specialist to determine if any special precautions need to be undertaken before starting exercise.

- *History of breathlessness with exercise or unusual chest pain:* These are obviously red flags for a potential heart problem, but they can be due to other factors such as indigestion, gastric reflux or muscular problems. A thorough check with your doctor will determine whether it is safe for you to commence a guided exercise program even in the presence of these conditions. Sometimes they may need to be more thoroughly investigated.

- *Being overweight or obese:* These are not exclusions for commencing an exercise program, but they may affect the choice of exercise that is undertaken. If you are significantly overweight or obese, you may have some mechanical disadvantages associated with weight bearing exercises and so need to be carefully guided through an appropriately prescribed exercise program. You not only will benefit with all the metabolic gains from this, but also should gradually reduce your weight through your increased calorie expenditure and better nutrition awareness.

- *Family history:* If you have a positive family history of ischaemic heart disease, diabetes, sudden death or other significant medical problems, these should also be discussed with your doctor to determine the impact they may have on an exercise program. In general, a regular exercise program will minimise or even eradicate the likelihood of developing these conditions if your lifestyle is suitably healthy. Nevertheless, it is important to recognise these in your family history and have the topic discussed.

- *Age over 40:* The exact age at which medical screening should be undertaken remains controversial (as discussed in chapter 5). Depending on the lifestyle you led through your 20s and 30s, some risk issues may emerge as you turn 40 and beyond — such as some of the medical conditions included in this list. If you're now over 40 and you have not had a recent medical check-up, booking one in with your GP is wise. This will give you and your GP some baseline information in relation to aspects such as your blood pressure, lipids and diabetes tendency, in order to help predict future problems. It will also assist with monitoring the impact that the planned exercise program has on these potential concerns.

- *Inactive for years:* Perhaps life pressures have stopped you doing any exercise for a long time. While many people were active at school, moving on to tertiary education, relationships, establishing careers and then family commitments often mean that exercise becomes a low priority during their 20s and 30s. If you feel you are in this group and significantly 'out of shape', it is important to have at least a brief discussion with your family doctor so that an appropriate lower intensity program can be initiated and gradually progressed to gain the health benefits going forward.

#4 Seek advice on planning your best exercise program
....

Finding the right exercise program for you and your current state of health is invaluable. Apart from having the appropriate health check-up with your doctor prior to commencing a program (see previous section) the other critical issue is just how to get started.

You have many options available. Some people will join a health club or gym, some will employ a personal trainer either in a group or private one-on-one format, while others will simply look online to determine the right exercise program for them.

I certainly advise that if you have any pre-existing medical conditions, have been sedentary for a while or are over 40, you should see your medical practitioner to make sure that it is okay to start the program. As mentioned, conditions such as high blood pressure, diabetes and high cholesterol may have an impact on your recommended type of exercise. In addition, your age, general state of fitness and other factors such as joint arthritis might affect your choice.

In more recent years, professionals such as exercise scientists or exercise physiologists working in the health industry can also help you with your exercise program. Finding the correct individual can be a challenge, but your family doctor or local physiotherapist may be able to advise you on individuals in your area who can assist with designing your program.

In any event, starting out at the appropriate level for you is important. From there, you can gradually progress, looking out for any signs of adverse effects such as muscle soreness or injury that may require some modifications to your program.

Unfortunately, I have had the experience of dealing with many individuals who were very enthusiastic at the start of their program, but did not seek the correct initial advice. They then became frustrated when they were injured and so lost motivation. Instead, seek out an individual who can set up the program appropriate for you so you are more likely to stay healthy and achieve the expected progress through a consistent approach. You don't want to end up in my office waiting room with your injury!

#5 Know how to start an exercise program

Throughout this book, I emphasise the need to have a regular and consistent exercise program in your lifestyle. Perhaps you're already undertaking an exercise program of some type, and perhaps that commitment is substantial. However, you might also be at the other end of the spectrum (and, seeing you're reading this book, I'm guessing that's more likely). If you're looking to start an exercise program, you need to be aware of some important considerations before you begin.

When starting an exercise program, it is important to find an activity that you enjoy and begin slowly with a gradual build-up. The easiest activity for many people to get started is a simple walking program on alternate days each week. While the ultimate target is 150 minutes per week of cardio (aerobic) activity, in the early days this amount can be less as you gradually build up your regular routine. Even a five-minute first attempt will get the habit started.

Once your exercise is established, you can start to build in a more varied and complete program. The three broad areas you need to consider are:

1. cardio (aerobic) activity

2.   strength (resistance) training

3.   flexibility and stretching.

Cardio (aerobic) activity

The aim here is to use large muscle groups in a consistent rhythmic manner. This can include walking, cycling, rowing, skipping, elliptical trainer, stair climber and running. Beginning at a slow intensity is important, ultimately building up to a moderate effort to gain further benefits. As you become fitter, you can add more intensity to your sessions, but certainly not at the beginning as you are starting out.

One simple method is to aim for a 10-minute walk on alternate days around your neighbourhood. After a week, you can build this up to 15 minutes, and then 20 minutes — with the ultimate aim of doing a minimum of 30 minutes on a five days per week basis (150 mins per week). You should aim for a moderate intensity where you can conduct a conversation with a workout buddy, but just be slightly breathless. You need to be able to talk, but not sing!

Strength training

Strength (resistance) training helps to build muscle tone, which not only assists with strength and posture, but also reduces fatigue and assists with preventing falls, and can aid balance, particularly as you move into the older age groups. However, the value of strength training is not only in building muscle tone. Many hormones and naturally occurring chemicals are released during strength and resistance training sessions. These agents have positive effects on a huge range of the body's metabolic processes, way beyond muscle improvement. These include both physical and mental health benefits.

Strength and resistance training has also been shown to assist with improvements in bone density, and some exciting studies of the last decade have shown important health benefits in a range of other conditions—such as cardiovascular health, diabetes, depression and other mental health issues, arthritis, certain cancers, and the prevention of gradual muscle decline (unkindly referred to as 'senile sarcopenia'), which occurs progressively in everyone. In fact, muscle strength declines by an average of 10 per cent per decade from the age of 30 years. However, by adding resistance training on a three times per week basis, you can minimise or even reverse the effect of this muscle strength decline. It is critical that this strength training be added to a balanced, complete exercise program. Your mind and body will thank you. And you don't have to be lifting really heavy weights to achieve these health benefits—they occur with modest efforts, and can even be gained through exercises that use your own body weight, such as squats, planks and lunges. How often do you need to commit to strength training? Completing two to three strength sessions each week, performing eight to 12 repetitions of each exercise, focusing on specific muscle groups and using correct form and technique, will get you there.

TIP
Be strong—strength matters for your physical and mental health.

Flexibility and stretching

As you age, your joints and the collagen and fascia tissue that binds your soft tissues together lose stretch and flexibility. A regular stretching program, which might be incorporated through activities such as yoga or Pilates, can assist with improving your joint range of motion. This also assists with improvements in your gait and helps you avoid the minor strains that can happen if you slip or move in an unexpected way when a joint is not used to the extreme movement. It is also helpful to have the flexibility to be able to reach down to put on your socks in the morning as you age!

FITT and HIIT

A good way to remember a simple acronym for a balanced cardio fitness program is the FITT principle. Here's how it works:

+ *Frequency:* Adding in four to five sessions per week of a consistent workout is the optimum. Some people will move up to doing seven days per week, but this is usually more in the realm of a competitive athlete.

+ *Intensity:* Starting at a moderate intensity is beneficial—this is where you're aiming an exertion rate of 6 to 7 out of 10, where 10 is your absolute maximum effort. If you can monitor your heart rate during activity—made easier with modern fitness watches—you should be looking at getting to 70 to 80 per cent of your maximum heart rate. (Maximum heart rate can be calculated as 220 minus your age, as a good general rule.)

+ *Type:* As mentioned, aerobic activity uses large muscle groups in a continuous rhythmic activity. What you choose (such as walking, cycling or rowing) doesn't matter, as long as you're working to improve cardiac output and blood flow to the body as well as the brain.

+ *Time:* Starting at a modest time of 10 minutes is fine if you are just beginning, but the ultimate aim is 30 minutes or more, five times per week. If you can do more than 30 minutes, you will gain extra health benefits.

(continued)

If you have any doubts about how to structure a FITT program, seek advice from your medical practitioner, a well-qualified personal trainer or an exercise physiologist skilled in exercise prescription.

As a bonus, and once you have your FITT program locked in, you may also add in some HIIT—or high intensity interval training. This is shorter bursts of exercise activity at much higher effort levels. This type of exercise has also been shown to improve many health and fitness parameters but has the advantage of needing less time. It does not suit everyone (and can have a higher risk of injury if you are just starting out) so you must seek advice on what type of exercise is right for your age, current fitness level and health situation.

#6 Understand what motivates you to improve your fitness

Why change at all? This is a valid question. Often, an individual needs to experience some sort of crisis before they make the changes needed to improve their health. This might take the form of a personal health event, such as a heart attack, or an event in the life of someone close to them—for example, a sibling or close friend with cancer, or losing someone through heart issues.

In my seminars over the years, I have collected responses from my audiences on what motivates them to change their health behaviour. Some are cheeky but all are relevant.

The most common are:

- a negative personal health event

- a negative event for a close friend, family member or colleague

- a health check-up that reveals an abnormal but correctable issue

- milestone birthday

- peer group pressure

- clothes not fitting

- retirement

- weight gain (embarrassment)

- job requirement

- vanity

- impending marriage

- recent divorce

- one of my seminars!

Do you recognise any of your motivations in the list of reasons? While some of them are humorous and somewhat tongue in cheek, many of them are easily identified with from a day-to-day perspective. Where do you sit? Are you taking responsibility? I hope I can convince you to act! Trust me — it's for your own good!

You will, of course, have other potential reasons to make a change for your better health. Uncover what these reasons are, and then use them to keep yourself motivated. Whatever it takes to motivate and continue to remind you to improve yourself is fine with me.

#7
....

Know your limits and keep exercise safe

Over the years, you may have heard of cases of tragic sudden deaths during exercising sessions. One highly prominent case was renowned cardiologist Dr Jim Fixx, who died in 1984 while out running. Dr Fixx was the author of the famous bestseller *The Complete Book of Running*—which had influenced tens of thousands of people to take up jogging and made him a guru of the running world. His death initially sent shockwaves through the running community and gave great voice to the opponents of exercise, who used his example to claim vigorous exercise was bad for you. I have personally had similar experiences of someone unexpectedly dying in my time as a race medical director or when part of a race medical care team for marathons, ocean swims and triathlons.

These events are shocking and extremely unfortunate. However, they are also extremely rare, and there is always an explanation.

Following a sudden tragic death occurring during exercise, an autopsy is almost always undertaken to determine the reason behind the death. In the majority of circumstances, a cardiac abnormality is detected—such as ischaemic heart disease (atherosclerosis), a genetic structural abnormality in the heart or an unusual abnormality that causes cardiac electrical rhythm disturbances known as 'arrhythmia'.

In many other circumstances, the individual who suffered an exercise-induced death will be found to have had significant lifestyle predisposing problems. These may not have been recognised or detected until the unfortunate incident, and can include coronary artery disease, hypertension, an abnormal lipid profile or another metabolic disorder that predisposed the individual to high risk of heart disease. Sadly, these generally are not detected early enough to allow for appropriate medical and lifestyle interventions prior to commencing a vigorous exercise program. Jim Fixx had a family history of heart disease, was a past heavy smoker and had been extremely overweight when younger. Unfortunately, his earlier poor lifestyle choices had predisposed him to cardiac disease.

This is another important reason why it is critical to undergo a thorough pre-participation medical clearance exam, especially if you have a family history of worrying medical conditions, such as a previous sudden death in a close relative.

By detecting these predisposing abnormalities, your doctor can prescribe an exercise program at an appropriate intensity. This can then minimise the risk of a negative event and, in fact, has the ability to help reduce some of the predisposing abnormalities such as high blood pressure, high cholesterol or coronary artery disease. (See earlier in this chapter for more information on medical screening before starting exercise.)

#8 Find time for exercise

When individuals find excuses as to why they don't look after their health or have a regular exercise program, one of the most common excuses given is, 'I don't have enough time.' Is this something that resonates with you?

As a busy professional myself, I sympathise with this perspective. We all have the same 168 hours available to us in any given week. How you spend that time is often determined by your occupation, family commitments, social activities, sleep and any other number of activities that tend to clog up your day-to-day lives. However, as Jean de la Bruyere observed back in 1688, 'Those who make the worst use of their time are the first to complain of its brevity.'

Do you realise that the recommended 150 minutes per week of regular exercise required to produce extraordinary health benefits represents only 1.5 per cent of your total available time in any given week? To me, this is a very small investment to make for an extremely large beneficial return. You are investing in your future in a massive way by putting aside the time for your health maintenance.

As a cartoon I regularly use in my seminars reads, 'What suits you more, spending 30 minutes per day exercising, or 24 hours a day dead?'

I have often said that those busy executives who do not find time for their health maintenance (usually males) will have a lot of time on their hands to contemplate their health situation when they are sitting in a coronary care unit, wired up to their heart monitor machines after experiencing a cardiac event such as a heart attack. Unfortunately, this is often the motivating event that prompts an individual to take action — if they are fortunate enough to survive the sudden cardiac event in the first place. (Unfortunately, many don't.)

> ## TIP
> Initially, as small a commitment as 60 minutes per week (15 minutes, four times a week) can begin the process of improving health profiles. The 150-minute target is something that can gradually be achieved as you progress through the program.

I understand that time is precious for all of us, but the whole point of this book is helping you extend the time you have to enjoy your life into your aging years. Investing a small amount of that time to achieve the overall goal seems to make a lot of sense. It is not something that can be acquired passively.

#9 Don't let excuses get in your way
....

I know many people, including my patients, who say they would like to do more exercise or be 'fitter', but they just don't get it done. Over the years I have heard just about all the excuses there are. The following are some of the more common excuses, along with my response:

- *'I am already in good health':* This is actually a very short-sighted perspective to take. Unfortunately, it will often take an adverse health event to change the mindset of this type of individual.

- *'I don't have time':* Yes, lack of time is a challenge for everyone. However, as mentioned in the previous section, we all have 168 hours in each week and committing the basic target of 150 minutes per week represents only 1.5 per cent of the total available time. This is a very small commitment to make for a huge return on health and quality of life. I repeat my earlier question: 'What suits you more, spending 30 minutes per day exercising, or 24 hours a day dead?'

- *'I dislike exercise – it's boring':* You have many options available as to the type of physical activity and exercise you can do. It is simply a matter of looking at the various options and finding an activity that is compatible with your time availability and things that you like to do. It does not need to be a one-dimensional approach. There is something for everyone.

- *'My health is too poor':* This is an interesting one. I understand that you may not be able to immediately embark on a moderately vigorous or even light exercise program due to a pre-existing medical condition. But you can seek a medical appointment with your health practitioner and discuss the options which are safe. Exercise has been shown to be beneficial for so many chronic illness conditions, and especially heart disease, cancers, diabetes and arthritis. Introducing an appropriate level of exercise (perhaps, for example, water-based hydrotherapy initially) and building slowly on this can assist greatly in the management of a problematic or chronic health condition. It is simply a matter of finding the best fit.

- *'I'm too tired/too lazy/too apathetic':* These ones annoy me! These excuses are obviously a mindset issue in some individuals. If you find yourself making these kinds of excuses, you need to have an honest counselling session with your health professional and fitness advisor in order to understand that the negative approach you're taking is not beneficial. You will likely benefit from having some psychological motivation and assistance, such as from a personal trainer or exercise prescription expert.

- *'I didn't know exercise was good for health':* My response? 'Where have you been?' It is hard to imagine that anyone could come up with this excuse in this day and age. Unfortunately, some people are still able to ignore the information and publicity that has been around for so many decades on the benefits of regular exercise in health promotion. If this is you, you're highly likely to benefit from reading this book and getting some advice on how to improve your health!

EXERCISE

- *'I can't afford to exercise':* Exercise does not need to be an expensive undertaking. You do not need to belong to an expensive health club or gym, or buy a bike, treadmill or other expensive equipment. Most people can get by with a pair of sports shoes and some comfortable clothing that they already have in their weekend wardrobe. Walking around the block in the fresh air and sunshine does not cost a great deal of money.

- *'My dog ate my running shoes/it's raining/cold outside (and so on)':* These individuals look for any lame excuse to get out of doing some exercise. Again, if this is you (and you can be honest and admit it), you will benefit from appropriate counselling and some simple encouragement that shows the benefits of getting out and beginning an exercise program, even at a very moderate or low level of intensity. You might even enjoy it enough to continue. The hardest part is making a start.

I'm sure you've heard—and made—many other excuses over the years. The point I'm making is simply that it is up to you to make the effort to start putting time into protecting your personal health. This means being organised and planning the week to invest in some personal health time.

#10 Start with small changes for big gains

You might be surprised at how small a change you need to make in your overall exercise program in order to gain initial health benefits. Simply going from doing nothing to doing as little as 60 minutes per week of walking or some other cardio exercise has been shown to reduce the overall risk of all causes of death by 25 per cent. This is a massive gain and is a far better outcome than any of the established pharmaceutical medications used to treat conditions such as high blood pressure or high cholesterol.

Progressing the 60 minutes per week up to a total of 150 minutes per week further reduces the all-cause mortality risk by 40 per cent — this is considered the sweet spot for optimal return of health benefits and reducing your risk of dying (known as 'all-cause mortality reduction'). Of course, some people do far more exercise than this and they can gain higher fitness benefits as they increase from moderate to more vigorous intensity exercise, but this is generally not required unless you are training for an event such as a marathon, fun run or other competition. (Of course, the choice is yours, based on your health and motivation to achieve higher levels of fitness.) Combining the cardio exercise time with some resistance (strength) training three times per week and some flexibility exercises will provide you with an optimal physical activity program.

#11 Take some time for recovery

Perhaps you're not surprised to hear that competitive athletes often train seven days per week, sometimes with multiple sessions per day. Their training program will vary depending on the type of sport they are undertaking, and of course these individuals are seeking high gains with their fitness and have a competitive goal in mind. Most individuals who are simply looking to get healthy and achieve modest level fitness benefits do not need this degree of frequency or intensity.

Indeed, this level of intensity can be dangerous — unless you are extremely fit, well-conditioned and somewhat genetically gifted, the likelihood of sustaining an injury with this type of training program is high. The concept of starting off slowly and building up gradually makes sense (as highlighted throughout this chapter). Even elite athletes have 'recovery' days to allow their bodies to gain maximum benefits from their training programs.

No hard and fast answer exists regarding how much exercise is too much. However, if you are getting excessive muscle soreness or sustaining injuries, you clearly need to re-evaluate the nature of the program and see what changes can be made to bring you back to a safer level. Like any medicine, a correct dose of exercise exists for you, free from side effects. Remember, the overall plan here is to improve your health, not provide you with another medical complaint!

So, yes, consistency is the key to improving, but you do not need to train like an athlete preparing for the next Olympics to make the progress. Giving yourself a recovery or rest day once or twice per week, and mixing up the type of exercises you do in order to spread the load around your body is a better way of ensuring you do not overstress and cause an injury or setback. Seek advice on an appropriately balanced program — and the right techniques — for your age and state of fitness and you will reap the benefits many times over.

#12 Prepare your workout clothes the night before

If you are an individual who prefers to do your exercise sessions first thing in the morning, you will be regularly tested, even with the best of intentions — either by inclement weather or simply through being tired from the activities from the day before. Getting yourself out from the warm bed to commit to your workout becomes a challenge, particularly if it's an outdoor session. Of course, having a workout friend you are meeting always helps because you have the added motivation of not wanting to feel guilty by letting them down if you don't turn up at your planned meeting spot or at an arranged meeting time.

However, one tip that I found particularly useful during my training time was to lay out my running clothes the night before so that they were easily accessible when I staggered out of bed in my half-awake state. By having my running top, shorts, socks and shoes neatly prepared the night before, I found it easier to get up, dress immediately in my outfit and head out the door. Once the session was underway, I was always grateful that I had made the effort to be prepared.

TIP

Regardless of the type of morning session you are planning, setting up the night before will help. Whether you're laying out your gym clothes, cycling gear, a running outfit or other clothing and equipment needed, just get organised ahead of time. It will be one less barrier to making the effort to get going on that next challenging morning session.

The range of modern apparel materials is fantastic these days so, if you can, treat yourself to some of the latest workout gear, so you feel great and comfortable. The protective gear available even for cold weather or rain conditions is so much better than in the past, so a little rain shower is no excuse for not getting out for your outdoor session. It's only water, folks!

#13 Increase your walking speed
....

I highlight throughout this book the value of regular exercise, particularly cardio or aerobic activities. Walking is the top of the list for most people when it comes to choosing an activity that is convenient, accessible and requires minimal equipment.

Walking is easy and convenient, but remember — speed matters. The speed at which you walk determines the amount of energy you are expending, and walking at a very slow speed does not provide much in the way of cardio benefits. Regardless of the aerobic activity you choose, the benefits are greater when the intensity of the activity is at moderate levels. As the intensity goes up, the fitness benefits improve, but this needs to be progressed over time.

Many studies have confirmed that the speed of walking determines the overall benefits. For people who walk at a naturally faster speed (my friends will tell you I am one of them), the gain is greater in health and fitness benefits and, therefore, this converts into a healthy anti-aging benefit. Walking at a faster space is associated with a reduction in the all-cause mortality risk I mention earlier in this chapter, especially for the common conditions such as cardiac disease. It has also been shown to reduce dementia risk. So although stopping to admire the neighbours' gardens and smell the roses while you are out walking is lovely, the real intention of the session is to gain fitness benefits, so you need to keep moving at a moderately vigorous pace (or build up to this pace) in order to achieve the results.

To really drive this home, in 2011 the *British Medical Journal* published a humorous article that uncovered the speed at which the 'Grim

Reaper'—representing death—walked. Those who wish to avoid death need to walk at a faster speed than death itself—calculated as 0.8 metre per sec (around 3 kilometres per hour). You need to keep ahead of this pace to stay alive!

'Walk away from your doctor' is another phrase I have used on many occasions in my seminars. This is not meant to alienate my medical colleagues, and hopefully the theme is obvious. If you keep yourself healthy, you are less likely to be unwell and need to visit your doctor. Walking provides this.

So next time you are planning a walk, either solo or with an exercise colleague, make sure that you add a reasonable pace to the walking (enough intensity to carry on a conversation, but not sing!) and you will be making yet another contribution to your overall health maintenance.

#14 Get those steps in

Many health professionals and exercise guidelines now recommend a target of 10 000 steps per day as a reasonable goal for health and fitness gains.

Is this necessary? And why 10 000? The origin of the 10 000 steps guideline dates back to the 1960s, when Japanese company Yamasa launched a commercial pedometer product with the name 'manpo-kei'—which literally translates as '10 000-step meter'. At the time, no scientific data existed to support this number of steps. Subsequently, many validated studies have looked at step counts as a way of monitoring exercise intensity and workload. And counting your steps is definitely an easy way to measure a workout—compared to, say, calorie expenditure or other more complex indicators of load.

What the studies did discover, however, is that you do not need to reach the total figure of 10 000 steps to achieve reasonable health benefits. In fact, multiple studies have shown that as few as 2500 steps convey health benefits. As you do more, the benefits do improve, with the sweet spot appearing to be around 7700 steps per day, as published by Harvard researcher Dr I- Min Lee in 2019. This study showed that benefits began to accumulate at 4700 steps per day and gradually increased up to a limit of around 10 000 steps per day. Benefits appeared to taper off above this number. For older women, the number of steps required to obtain health benefits is even fewer. Good news ladies!

The message is quite straightforward. Aim for a step count in the optimal range of 7000 to 9000 steps per day to achieve the health benefits related to a walking program. Even at 4000 to 5000 steps per day, you are adding to your health profile. The intensity of the walking speed is also relevant, as discussed in the previous section.

#15 Boost your mitochondria

Mitochondria are very specialised cells in the body that help convert food into energy for body metabolism. They are often known as the 'powerhouses' of the body's cells. Mitochondria are responsible for generating a compound called adenosine triphosphate (ATP), the main energy component for your body's cells. They help cells to communicate between each other and also monitor cell breakdown and cell death (a process known as 'apoptosis'), particularly during aging. Clearly, having healthy mitochondria is important, particularly as you get into your advancing years. In fact, the health of your mitochondria is critical in determining how quickly you age. Mitochondrial dysfunction is one key hallmark of aging and leads to decline in both skeletal muscle and brain (central nervous system) function.

Mitochondria contain a component of your DNA in each of their cells. As you are no doubt aware, your DNA determines much of your health status on many levels, and provides direction to many of your body's metabolic processes to help maintain optimal health. At a basic level, mitochondria influence how your genes function. (I remember when I was in second year medical school and training regularly as a middle-distance runner. At that stage, I was on the cusp of making the Australian running team and was known for doing lots of training sessions, occasionally making me late for of my med school classes! One of my medical classmates, Anthony Baird, made a comment to me that has stuck with me to this day. He said, 'Peter, your mitochondria must be the size of footballs.' At that time, I did not appreciate the role of mitochondria in overall body function and energy production, but it just goes to show that Anthony was a much brighter student than me in my physiology class!)

Some of the important roles that mitochondria have in keeping us healthy include the following:

- *Energy production:* As just mentioned, ATP is primarily produced in mitochondria as a way of powering the body's cellular metabolic processes. The food you eat is converted into energy through an oxidative process known as the 'citric acid cycle' or 'Krebs cycle', and mitochondria play a vital role in this.

- *Cellular health and breakdown:* As cells age, they undergo apoptosis, a dying process. This clearly makes them less functional, and mitochondria play an extremely important role in helping to control the apoptosis process in the body. For example, in certain diseases such as cancer, the normal cellular breakdown becomes dysfunctional. Having mitochondria at optimal function is important in order to help control this process, particularly with certain degenerative diseases and these types of cancer.

- *Calcium storage:* Calcium is a vital mineral nutrient in your body, and is associated with many of the body's functions. It helps nerves function at optimal level, and is intimately involved in muscle and bone metabolism and the blood clotting processes. Mitochondria play a vital role in helping the body absorb calcium ions and store them until they are required by the body's metabolic processes.

- *Heat production:* Our body is capable of producing heat in a number of ways — through exercise, shivering and other mechanisms. Mitochondria are so clever that they can generate heat on their own without the shivering process.

Unfortunately, mitochondria can be damaged or suffer disease processes in many ways. When your mitochondria do not function at optimal level, a range of illnesses may follow, including the following:

- chronic fatigue

- diabetes

- gastrointestinal problems

- heart, liver or kidney disease

- mental health disorders

- muscle weakness

- neurological problems, including dementia.

So how do you protect your mitochondria?

The health of our mitochondria reflects the overall way you protect the health of your body. Looking after your mitochondria is essential to our overall goal of healthy living into old age (even though they are too small to see!). Through regular exercise, good nutrition and controlling your oxidative stress levels, your mitochondria can remain functional. (See chapter 7 for more on nutrition and chapter 9 for more on stress management.)

Unhealthy living choices inhibit mitochondrial performance, reducing their ability to function well in controlling the aging processes in our body. While their exact role in the anti-aging process is still being researched, it is important that you follow the principles of healthy living to boost your mitochondria — and hopefully you too will be on the pathway to having mitochondria as big as footballs!

#16 Increase your NAD

In recent times, some of the anti-aging research been focused on a compound known as NAD. NAD stands for nicotinamide adenine dinucleotide, and it is a central mediator of cellular energy and a crucial link between your nutritional intake, health and effective cellular metabolism.

NAD plays an important role in assisting the body to work effectively, including having a positive effect on mitochondrial function and boosting ATP production essential for energy and exercise. (See the previous section for more on mitochondria and ATP production.)

NAD also plays an important role in limiting oxidative stress as a result of normal daily body functions. Production of NAD declines with age and a deficiency may be linked to accelerated aging in vulnerable individuals.

You obtain NAD in your diet through ingestion of the essential amino acid tryptophan, which is found in fish such as salmon, tuna and sardines, and in certain types of mushrooms. You can also purchase NAD supplements to be taken orally. From my perspective, obtaining your nutrient intake through healthy natural food choices rather than manufactured supplements is always best, but you should seek advice from your own doctor.

#17 Increase your lifespan — and healthspan — with exercise

Ever since I began in medical practice, I have encouraged my patients to be active and develop an exercise program compatible with their lifestyle. Benefits such as weight control, improved self-esteem and increased energy appeal to everyone. Previously, and as mentioned in chapter 1, I have told my patients, 'Exercise may not make you live a day longer, but you will live a longer day.' Well, things have changed. I can say to my patients that evidence now shows that regular moderate-level exercise can actually help them live longer. What a bonus!

The main cause of death in Australia is heart disease. The risk factors for this are well documented, and include high blood pressure, smoking, elevated lipids (especially bad LDL cholesterol), obesity and diabetes. These all significantly magnify the risk of developing heart disease prematurely. Even those who survive into older age with these types of risk factors and diseases will find the morbidity of their illness has a major impact on reducing their quality of life. Wouldn't it be great to reduce this morbidity and poor quality of life so that, as our medical knowledge increases to allow us to live a longer life, we are also able to live a healthier and more productive life in those extra years?

Regular physical activity has been shown undisputedly to have a beneficial effect on the risk factors linked to poor health, particularly ischaemic heart disease. This benefit occurs regardless of whether the physical activity is in the form of a structured exercise program or simply a lifestyle pattern that includes some form of physical exertion during the normal course of the day. Benefits include lower blood pressure, lower cholesterol, weight reduction, reduced risk of diabetes, less osteoporosis and reduction in stress and some types of cancer. However, research now suggests exercise may also have an independent and direct effect on health, rather than only achieving the indirect benefits just mentioned.

Many studies also show that physiological improvements can be obtained through regular physical activity, regardless of the age of the participant. For instance, an active 65 year old can perform at the same level as a sedentary 25 year old when measurements such as aerobic (oxygen) capacity are compared. In other words, the 'physiological age' of an individual can be considerably lower than their chronological age. Exercise appears to delay the effects of aging and many of the reduced performance parameters of an older individual previously (and often humorously) considered to be inevitable due to 'old age'.

Recent interest, and certainly one of the more controversial areas of research, has also focused on whether regular exercise can actually reverse the established disease processes, particularly those linked with heart disease. People with coronary artery disease, for example, who are placed on a regular exercise program have been shown to be able to achieve a reversal of the severity of the disease as measured by coronary angiography. (An angiogram is a highly specialised imaging X-ray that shows the health of the heart's blood vessels.) This knowledge has created great excitement among those concerned with managing heart disease patients and should encourage all individuals to seek advice on exercise regardless of their age or health status. Studies have shown for quite some time that an individual who exercises regularly is more likely to survive a heart problem, even a heart attack, simply because they have a stronger heart with a better blood supply than a non-exercising individual. Thus a fit person not only has less chance of experiencing illness such as heart disease, but also has a higher change of surviving a significant heart problem should it occur.

Without doubt, further long-range studies are required to establish the complex relationships between physical activity, physical fitness, disease prevention and health. One powerful study is the long-running Harvard alumni health study, started by Professor Ralph Paffenbarger in 1962. Although the study focused only on male Harvard graduates, its findings are still significant — including a markedly significant reduction in deaths from *all causes* in those individuals who had been active in their younger life and remained active into their later years. Those individuals who maintained a commitment to a fitness program not only lived longer, but also lived healthier than their less fit counterparts.

Finally, exercise has tremendous advantages over other methods of health promotion and risk reduction — exercise requires no drugs or surgery, is inexpensive and relatively painless, and requires no elaborate equipment. All it needs is your commitment and time — and time is something you will have in abundance when you live a longer, healthier life!

7

Nutrition

Nutrition is a major component of a healthy living plan. Food is life, and a healthy eating plan is essential for a long and happy one. Note that I'm not using the term 'diet plan' here. I don't like this term, because it implies some form of deprivation or unpleasant sacrifice. That's not my idea of the way to enjoy a healthy life experience!

Eating is an everyday event we often take for granted. You've likely had a memorable meal on a special occasion or at a favourite restaurant. However, have you stopped to think of the role that healthy nutrition plays in overall health maintenance and lifestyle performance?

I can't recall the first time I heard the phrase, 'You are what you eat.' (I do remember a humorous response from one individual: 'I need to eat a skinny person!') But it's true that healthy food makes a difference to the performance of your body.

Your body requires a range of fuels for its metabolism. The healthier the fuel you provide, the more likely the metabolic processes will occur in an efficient and optimal manner.

Food—a critical component of healthy living

No doubt you're aware that Australia and the world has been undergoing an obesity crisis over recent decades. The link between obesity and poor health is well established, and is associated with much more than simply being overweight—it is linked to heart disease, diabetes, some cancers and lack of physical fitness. The type of fuel you provide to your body determines how efficiently it performs. Can you imagine supplying a Formula One racing car with two-stroke lawnmower fuel? You wouldn't expect to get great performance in that circumstance. Similarly, your body requires appropriate high-octane fuel to perform at its best.

Unfortunately, we live in a world of fast food—full of preservatives and artificial colouring, and high in salt and sugar. While this is often known as 'convenience food', it has also been shown to be a source of obesity, lethargy and poor performance in life.

Most athletes are aware of the correct nutrition to obtain optimal performance in whatever sport they pursue. There is no reason why you shouldn't also be looking for optimal performance in your everyday life by using similar nutrition principles. This chapter shows you how.

#18 Focus on your gut health

To appreciate why great nutrition adds to our healthy living, understanding how the gastrointestinal (GI) tract works and why you need to keep your gut healthy is useful. Your gut and digestive system is critical in optimising the role of diet and nutrition in enhancing your health.

Structure of the digestive tract

Your digestive tract (or gut) is an extremely delicate and important organ system in your body. It is made up of multiple segments, beginning with the mouth and oral cavity and finishing up with the rectum. Along the way are the oesophagus, duodenum, stomach, small bowel, and large bowel, also known as the colon. This digestive tract is supported by important organs such as the pancreas, gall bladder and liver.

The gut can be up to 10 metres in length and contains millions of cells and multiple digestive enzymes to assist with the proper absorption of food. In addition, the gut contains over 500 varieties of bacteria, which are essential for body health and correct food absorption. The transit time of food through your digestive system varies between 24 and 72 hours, depending on the nature of the food ingested and your normal microbiome system.

On top of all that, a system known as the 'gut–brain axis' allows the digestive system to provide essential information to the brain in relation to your body's function. For instance, the gut is involved in the production of a chemical hormone called serotonin, which is essential for your mental stability and is often referred to as the 'happy hormone'. (See chapter 8 for more on serotonin.)

The gut microbiome

Your gut lining is teeming with live organisms to assist with digestion — known collectively as the 'gut microbiome'. Scientists estimate that the human genome contains over 23 000 genes and hundreds of trillions of biomes. Biomes are present in many areas of the body, including the oral cavity, respiratory system, skin, urinary tract and gut.

The microbes in your gut play an important role in the absorption of protein, starch, mucous, sugars and polysaccharides. A healthy gut microbiome allows you to gain maximum benefit from the foods you eat and sets you up for a much healthier future. A healthy gut microbiome can help support immune, heart and brain health, and may help control blood sugar and lower the risk of diabetes. Good microbes in your gut can even have anti-inflammatory effects.

What you eat plays a major role in the make-up of your gut microbiome. As mentioned, the idea that 'you are what you eat' has been around for a while, and research is now emerging that highlights your ability to personalise your nutritional plan to optimise health and the behaviour of your gut microbiome. This research may lead to you being able to develop a personalised 'nutrition plan' that is best suited to your own genetics and metabolism to boost your gut health, and so boost your overall health.

Breeding good bacteria

The mention of the word the word 'bacteria' tends to immediately conjure up a sense of something nasty or a problem in the body. However, many types of healthy bacteria in the body play an important role in maintaining body metabolism. These good bacteria are particularly important in the gut, but are also needed in other areas such as the oral cavity and even on the largest organ in the body — our skin surface.

By following good personal hygiene practices and a well-balanced healthy eating plan, you can ensure that your body's good bacteria remain at an optimal level. This is particularly important for the lining of your digestive system, where the gut microbiome is such an important component of a healthy body's overall metabolic environment.

A diet that includes natural fermented foods and fibre from colourful fruits and vegetables is a great way to start — as is picking up some of the tips throughout this chapter. Having healthy sleep habits and managing stress levels (see chapters 8 and 9) are other ways to support a healthy gut.

#19 Know the fuel your body needs

The correct intake of fuel provides your body with optimal ingredients to provide you with a healthy gut environment and energy for your lifestyle. Over the years, you may have read and seen conflicting articles in relation to how an ideal diet should be structured relative to the percentage contribution of starchy foods (carbohydrates), fatty foods, protein, and other components such as vitamins and minerals.

In recent decades, you have likely also seen plate sizes and portion sizes increase dramatically, particularly in countries such as the United States. This has resulted in the problem of 'portion distortion', which in turn has meant increased kilojoule (calorie) intake, well above that needed for day-to-day maintenance. Products such as 'triple-cheese double-bacon burgers' with upsized side orders of sugary soda drinks and salted chips have been a staple diet for many years in some households. The advertising is particularly directed at young children and adolescents. We all need to get back to the basics of healthy, organically grown fruit and vegetables to allow us to offset the damage caused by highly processed foods which not only contribute to poor nutrition, but also increase the risk of inflammation. (See action 21, 'Choose foods that are best for your brain and body', for more on inflammation.)

A varied diet of vegetables, fruit and lean protein together with adequate fluid intake and exercise is easy to achieve once you get into good habits. This will assist in providing you with the ideal program

NUTRITION

to maximise your energy needs and promote healthy living together with anti-aging processes.

The best diet contains naturally produced foods, free from preservatives and heavy processing. The body has adapted over many thousands of years to being able to extract the best vitamins, minerals and nutrients from natural food supplied to it.

Finally, remember that having an occasional 'treat' day, where you might stray from the general advice provided here, is fine. (We are all human!) But be aware of the price to pay afterwards, and needing to make up for your treat day at other times with the majority of your eating plan following my nutritional guidelines for a healthy gut. (It's no longer a treat if you have it every day!)

#20 Balance your food intake for body and brain

A well-planned diet for day-to-day living comprises a blend of healthy carbohydrates, lean protein and healthy fats, together with essential vitamins and minerals. I do not want to specify an exact percentage of each major component because this can vary depending on individual needs. Factors such as age, occupation, activity level and current health status can all influence and determine the make-up of your diet. A medical practitioner or accredited dietitian or nutritionist can advise you on this more accurately.

In the simplest terms, carbohydrates and fats provide the energy for your metabolism, while the protein foods provide the building blocks for tissue maintenance and recovery. You need a certain level of healthy fats in your diet to maintain energy levels, assist metabolism and help in the production of various hormones.

For basic day-to-day function, males require an average of 1500 calories per day. For females, it is slightly less at an average of 1200 calories per day. Remember—these are just averages. If you have a very active lifestyle (including exercise), you will require more calories proportional to your level of exertion. I know some athletes who consume between 7000 and 8000 calories in a single day—but they are using that fuel for their high intensity training and competition times.

When cooking for yourself and/or your family, develop some basic recipes—for example, wok stir-fry dishes and pasta with low-fat chicken, beef, vegetarian or seafood sauces. If you eat meat, grill a lean steak once a week with a healthy green salad on the side. (Grilled tofu, with some lentils or beans added to the salad, is a great plant-based alternative.) Avoid complicated rich sauces or anything deep fried. Occasional takeaway is fine—again, avoid the fried stuff.

Finally, the need for adequate water intake cannot be overemphasised—see 'Good fluid intake and hydration', later in this chapter, for more.

NUTRITION

> ### *TIP*
> Feed your body and brain well and you will be on the right path to achieving progress in your personal and work life. If you follow my healthy living advice tips in this book and head towards that '100 and beyond' target, you will certainly want your brain to be functioning at its best!

Eat most/plenty/regularly/less

The following is a simplified general food guide for what you should eat:

+ *Eat most:* Vegetables (fresh or snap frozen), fruit and water.

+ *Eat plenty:* Healthy protein, fish, chicken, turkey, tofu, lentils, beans and salads.

+ *Eat regularly:* Lean red meat, multigrain breads, pasta, rice, low-fat dairy products (yoghurt, cheese and milk).

+ *Eat less:* Sweet biscuits, cakes, processed and refined carbohydrate foods, high-fat snacks (chips, crackers), anything fried, most takeaway foods, caffeine 'booster 'drinks.

#21 Choose foods that are best for your brain and body

Certain foods are particularly beneficial to the important systems in our body. The following sections outline what they are. Once you learn how readily available these foods are, you will be able to choose wisely, more easily. Your body will thank you!

Food for your brain

Your brain needs proper fuel and energy for it to function properly. Your brain gets its main energy supply from glucose, and this is therefore its preferred source of fuel. As a young medical student, I remember being taught that the body has an in-built mechanism for protecting brain fuel supply. Even in your most malnourished state, the body holds a supply of glucose in reserve (especially in your liver) to allow the brain to keep you alive until the very end of your body's fuel reserves. So, the brain is obviously the body's favourite organ — and rightly so!

In many ways, the brain is also the most important organ in the body (although the gut may disagree with that). Optimal brain function obviously improves your mental performance and cognitive skills, and protecting your brain reduces your risk of developing some of the common disorders such as dementia, Parkinson's disease or Alzheimer's disease.

Apart from the obvious need for glucose to provide energy, some evidence also suggests that omega-3 fatty acids (oils) assist with brain nutrition and function. In addition, B vitamins contribute to improved mental performance and mood. Some studies suggest choline (often grouped with the B vitamins) can assist with improved memory and reaction times, and reduced fatigue. The active ingredient in turmeric, curcumin, has been shown to have benefits for your body and brain, including reducing the risk of depression and Alzheimer's disease.

All this means is that, if you manage to feed your brain well, you will improve function such as concentration, motivation, memory and reaction time, reduce stress and maybe even slow down the process of brain aging! That's another step in my plan for you to age 'youthfully'.

The foods that can be particularly beneficial for brain health include:

- blueberries

- broccoli

- coffee

- dark chocolate

- eggs

- fatty fish high in omega-3 oils — salmon, swordfish, cold-water fish

- green tea

- nuts

- oranges

- pumpkin seeds

- turmeric.

Food for your heart

Clearly the heart is also a very important organ in the body. Heart health depends on several components, including exercise, good cardiac blood supply and healthy heart muscle. Foods that have been associated with a healthy heart include:

- avocado

- beans

- berries

- dark chocolate

- fatty fish high in omega-3 oils

- garlic

- green leafy vegetables

- green tea

- olive oil (extra virgin)

- tomatoes

- walnuts

- whole grains.

Foods to boost the immune system

Immunity is such an important part of your defence against infection. This has been particularly brought to everyone's attention since 2020 with the COVID-19 pandemic, which ravaged the world, affecting global economies and causing tragic deaths in so many individuals. The ability to fight infection is associated with a highly functioning immune system. People who exercise regularly boost their immune system, but certain foods have also been associated with enhancing the body's immune response.

These foods include:

- almonds

- broccoli

- citrus fruits

- garlic

- ginger

- green tea

- kiwi fruit

- papaya

- poultry

- red peppers

- shellfish — lobster, oysters

- spinach

- sunflower seeds

- turmeric

- yoghurt.

Foods to fight inflammation

Inflammation has traditionally been associated with conditions such as painful joints or skin surface lesions. Pain, redness and the angry appearance of the affected tissue are all associated with the inflammation process. However, in recent decades an extensive amount of research has looked at the role that general body inflammation plays in ill health. This form of inflammation is often invisible on the surface but has a major impact on overall health. Generalised inflammation has been associated with heart disease, diabetes, stroke and certain cancers, and in aggravating underlying orthopaedic and musculoskeletal diseases such as rheumatoid arthritis. High inflammation levels in your system are now acknowledged as a cause of more rapid aging. The new term 'inflammaging' is aptly used to describe the adverse outcome.

While the debate continues about the role of some dietary foods in promoting inflammation, current research suggests that certain foods are extremely important in helping the body to minimise inflammation tendencies. These foods include:

- berries — strawberries, blueberries

- citrus fruits

- fatty fish (omega 3 oils)

- green leafy vegetables

- nuts

- olive oil

- tomatoes.

#22 Avoid processed foods
....

Avoiding processed foods is critical, because these promote inflammation in many individuals. Processed foods often contain nitrates, tartrate, salt, preservatives and hidden sugars, which can be disguised under many different names. In many processed convenience foods, the hidden sugar is often labelled as 'corn syrup', 'dextrose', 'fructose' or 'rice syrup'.

Be wary of these highly processed ingredients when choosing foods to promote good health and minimise inflammation tendency. (Refer to the previous section for foods that fight inflammation.)

As someone who spent my early years on a rural property, I had the advantage of eating foods that were pretty much all grown in our own garden. Fresh vegetables and fruit together with protein such as beef, chicken, rabbit and duck were all staple parts of my everyday diet as a youngster and young athlete. My grandmother used to have a saying: 'If I didn't grow it, pick it or shoot it, it must be processed!' These days, she would probably be right in most circumstances, given the highly mass-produced foods that are available now at so many of our supermarkets.

There is no short cut to healthy nutrition. It cannot be obtained through taking a pill or supplement from a health food store. Choosing healthy foods from a range of colourful fruits and vegetables will ensure that you obtain the natural ingredients and so help ensure your gut microbiome functions at maximal performance.

#23 Focus on good carbohydrates

In recent times, we have seen a heightened focus on excessive carbohydrate intake and how this might contribute to the obesity crisis. Carbohydrates include foods such as bread, rice, pasta, potatoes and other starchy foods. These foods are the immediate source of glucose for energy in the body and are, of course, essential for our existence. Excessive carbohydrates will only be stored as useless fat (which I call 'ballast') if they are not consumed as a fuel.

Yes, some carbohydrates are bad for you. The market is full of highly processed carbs that contain hidden preservatives and can be higher in sugar and lower in fibre than the ideal carbohydrates we need for energy. These foods are known to have a high *glycaemic index*. 'Glycaemic index' is a term referring to the rate at which the blood sugar level rises following ingestion of a carbohydrate product. Foods with a high glycaemic index are broken down quickly in the body and produce a spike in the blood sugar (glucose level), which then results in high insulin demand from the pancreas gland, followed by a 'crash' in blood sugar level, making us feel unsatisfied or lethargic.

Bad carbohydrates, such as highly processed white bread, muffins, doughnuts, cakes, cookies, potato chips and other 'convenience snacks' are all too readily available and are also a cause for concern.

However, healthy carbohydrates are readily available, such as grains, fresh vegetables (especially when eaten raw), certain fruits, wholemeal pasta, and healthy grain breads as well as oatmeal, legumes and barley—all of which have a low glycaemic index, resulting in a gradual release of energy throughout the day. This means they provide a more sustained and satisfying outcome after being ingested, and are less likely to cause the lethargy that often follows the rapid satisfaction achieved through poor carbohydrate intake. These low-GI carbs are a great source of your daily energy.

These 'good carbohydrates' also help to stabilise blood glucose levels and allow your pancreas to function more efficiently. This leads to more stable insulin levels and avoids the problem of *low insulin sensitivity*, a common condition where the body does not respond well to changing blood sugar levels, and *insulin resistance*, which is a precursor of diabetes.

#24 Build and repair with protein

Protein provides the essential building blocks for your body. Proteins are made up of chains of amino acids, which are found in every cell in our body. They are critical for cell repair and regeneration at all stages of life, and especially during childhood and pregnancy. Proteins are also required for muscle recovery after exercise.

Guidelines vary as to the amount of protein you need in your diet, but most nutrition experts recommend an intake of around 15 to 35 per cent of your total calories. (One gram of protein is equivalent to four calories.) Your specific requirements for protein intake depend on many factors, including your body type, activity levels and age. A good guideline is to average around 2 to 3 grams of protein per kilogram of body weight each day. Some athletes will increase their protein intake in the hope of providing additional repair for their muscles, but it is important to monitor protein intake so as not to overload kidney function.

Good sources of amino acids (proteins) in food include meat, milk, fish, eggs and chicken. Amino acids are also found in tofu, beans, nuts, legumes, and some grains.

In combination with carbohydrate intake and healthy fat intake, protein is one component of the important trio of nutrients to maintain optimal body health.

Make sure you choose healthy sources of protein for your shopping cart, and you will be taking further steps for excellent body maintenance. In particular, you'll be helping to offset the decline in muscle function that does occur as we age through the decades beyond 40. This process (known as muscle 'sarcopenia'—refer to the previous chapter) can be slowed through appropriate training, including strength training, together with adequate protein in the diet, helping you maintain good body shape, balance and tone.

#25 Know your good fats and bad fats

Fat intake in our everyday diet is often the subject of significant criticism. However, distinguishing between good fats and bad fats is important. Fat is essential in our diet — it is the type of fat you eat that requires an understanding and wise choices.

The 'good fats' (healthy fats) are necessary and beneficial for body health and maintenance of metabolic balance. Good fats need to be included in any well-designed diet and include *monounsaturated* and *polyunsaturated* fats. Sources of these types of fats are olive, canola, sunflower and avocado oils, as well as nuts, seeds and any oily fish that is rich in omega-3 oils (which includes salmon and tuna).

The 'bad fats' (unhealthy fats) are known as 'trans fats'. These are common in processed foods that use hydrogenated oil. These fats are known to increase the low-density lipoprotein (LDL — 'bad') cholesterol in the lipid system and contribute to many of the cardiovascular diseases.

The final type of fat you need to understand is *saturated* fats. These are not as bad as trans fats but need to be taken in moderation. They are found in natural butter, cheese, ice cream and high-fat red meats. They are also contained in coconut and palm oils. Used in small amounts, they can add variety and flavour in meals without contributing to an increase in significant lipid dysfunction.

Many people try to choose low-fat foods in the belief that they are healthier. Unfortunately, many manufacturers replace the fat in these foods with sugar, salt or other additives to provide better palatability. This, of course, adds additional calories and is certainly not a healthy way to achieve weight loss. You can lose weight on a fat-containing diet, provided you have a good balance of all nutrients.

Make yourself familiar with the good fats and bad fats so you're more knowledgeable when choosing appropriate foods for your shopping cart.

NUTRITION

#26 Cut your
.... sugar

'Sugar is great for energy' is a phrase that was frequently put to me as a youngster, and perhaps you have also heard it. At one stage, I probably even thought that white sugar was the greatest source of nutritional energy that I could have as a performance athlete. How wrong I was!

Sugar (in the form of glucose) is a primary source of fuel for our body, and particularly our muscles. However, the manner in which it is consumed or delivered to our bodies has been more thoroughly studied now than ever in the past. The end result of all this focus may surprise you — in that excessive intake of sugar has become one of the biggest challenges in overcoming poor nutrition habits (and tackling obesity) in society today.

The consumption of plain sugar can result in a very rapid rise in the blood sugar (glucose) level and provide a definite rapid 'energy hit'. However, for the body to deal with this sugar load, insulin needs to be released from the pancreas so that the sugar can be taken up by the various organs, including the muscles, and efficiently utilised for energy. This insulin surge can result in a metabolic event known as 'crashing', where the blood sugar level subsequently drops quite rapidly, often bringing on a sense of fatigue and lethargy as a result.

As discussed, foods that have a high glycaemic index (such as processed carbohydrates, white bread and pasta) result in a similar rapid release of glucose into the bloodstream, and so increased need for insulin to be released by the pancreas. This is why low glycaemic index foods should form a major component of good nutrition practices to provide energy throughout the course of the day.

However, these carbohydrate foods need to be balanced out with other sources of energy, such as healthy fats, to provide a more sustained metabolic balance and to avoid your insulin system being overloaded. The aim is to avoid a situation of insulin resistance or low insulin sensitivity, both of which are precursors of diabetes, one of the major metabolic conditions you should be trying to minimise. (See the nearby breakout box for more on the connection between insulin and diabetes.)

As I've mentioned, much of the food I consumed as a youngster was grown on our small rural property, meaning I was lucky enough to have high-quality nutrition with unprocessed natural foods in abundance. Nevertheless, I still remember my father enjoying his tea black and strong with two heaped teaspoons of white sugar as part of his daily ritual. In my very early days of drinking tea, I followed my father's lead and added sugar, but have since weaned myself off this as my palate and nutrition knowledge has expanded.

So, what is the bottom-line message?

Am I advocating that you should avoid sugar completely? Certainly not. However, the addition of sugar to cooking and other foods in your day-to-day life is something you really need to reconsider and minimise. Save sugar for occasional use only. Appealing sweets such as cakes, cookies and other dessert type foods also are very high in sugar content and, again, should only be eaten as an occasional treat. Make sure they do not make up a large component of your weekly nutrition plan.

In addition, it is important to have a look at food labels when buying pre-prepared and processed 'convenience foods', because 'hidden sugars' are often included in their ingredients. Terms such as 'corn syrup', 'dextrose', 'sucrose', 'fructose' are all alternative names for sugar, and many of the heavily processed products available contain these. Eating these foods adds to the sugar load in your day-to-day or weekly consumption, and creates extra stress for your pancreas as it produces insulin to deal with the sugar absorption and utilisation.

Sugars that are unable to be utilised immediately are generally converted into fat for subsequent storage, leading to weight gain and obesity. So while the treats may be occasionally justified, make sure you don't overlook the healthier components of your nutrition plan to assist with better metabolic stabilisation and looking after your body's energy and repair processes.

The connection between insulin and diabetes

Insulin is an essential hormone produced by the pancreas gland. It plays a critical role in controlling the blood glucose level in your body and allowing for the uptake of glucose into the body's metabolic pathways. Without insulin, the glucose produced from the food you eat to provide energy could not be delivered to your muscles and other important organs such as the brain, liver and kidney.

Those individuals who do not produce their own insulin or have insulin that is not working effectively suffer from the condition known as 'diabetes'. When insulin does not allow glucose to be moved into the body's tissues and organs, glucose builds up in the bloodstream, known as 'hyperglycaemia'.

Type 1 diabetes occurs when individuals are born with a condition where the pancreas does not produce enough insulin and these individuals usually require daily injections of insulin to control their blood sugar.

Type 2 diabetes can occur later in life when the pancreas slows down and does not produce enough insulin or when other lifestyle factors contribute to a condition known as 'insulin resistance'. In these individuals, the insulin they produce is no longer effective at keeping the blood glucose level under control. Insulin levels can also rise in an attempt to cope, but the body cannot efficiently utilise the glucose consumed. Measuring insulin levels in the blood should be part of a thorough health check-up, and abnormal levels can indicate impending diabetes.

This second type of diabetes (also referred to 'lifestyle diabetes') is generally associated with other metabolic problems such as obesity, high blood pressure and lack of fitness. It can be managed with exercise, weight loss and lifestyle changes. In some cases, medications can be used to help lower blood glucose levels.

Uncontrolled diabetes is a major health issue that affects many body systems, including the heart, kidney, nervous system and eyesight.

Yet again, exercise can be therapeutic, with research showing that blood glucose levels are lowered during and after activity, reducing the risk of diabetes complications.

NUTRITION

#27 Eat some chocolate!

Chocolate as a health supplement? I've got to be kidding, right? Chocolate in its most basic form is often a focus of much criticism in relation to poor nutrient value and potential high sugar content. However, chocolate contains many health-promoting nutrients and has been shown to reduce the risk of heart disease when taken in moderate amounts. Chocolate is rich in antioxidants, which are important for body health — in fact, chocolate has a higher content of antioxidants than many traditional foods.

Chocolate, particularly dark chocolate, has been discussed for many years as a potential healthy food source. Indeed, the concept of a good glass of red wine with some dark Belgian chocolate appeals to many people (myself included ... and many of my friends).

The health benefits really depend on what type of chocolate you're considering. The cocoa content of the chocolate needs to be between 70 and 85 per cent for you to gain the best health benefits. This results in a darker chocolate, which despite having some calories, does have less sugar than other varieties. Dark chocolate also contains fibre, iron, magnesium, potassium, zinc and selenium, all important ingredients in body health. Health food! Who would have thought?

Yes, chocolate also contains fats, but these are healthy fats, particularly oleic acid, a monounsaturated fat, found in healthy olive oils. Chocolate may also contain small amounts of caffeine, but less so than coffee.

Chocolate has also been shown to contain polyphenols, which are associated with positive benefits on the body's metabolic functions. Polyphenols have been shown to reduce LDL (bad) cholesterol and result in an overall benefit of lowering lipid levels.

So how much can you eat? Studies have shown that eating around 40 to 50 grams of chocolate per week can reduce the risk of disease, particularly heart disease, by a modest 9 per cent. Unfortunately, eating greater amounts beyond 100 grams per week does not seem to be associated with the same health benefits.

It is, of course, important to look at chocolate consumption in moderation. But adding some high-quality (at least 70 per cent cocoa content) dark chocolate to your shopping cart, along with other healthy snacks such as berries and nuts, means you can enjoy life, but still be contributing to a healthy lifestyle. Happy shopping!

#28 Use salt sparingly

Salt is another of those components of Western diets that attracts a lot of publicity—usually as being an unhealthy ingredient. You might be surprised at how much salt you consume during the day, even if you do not add salt to any of your foods or cooking. It is already a component of many of the foods available, and particularly if you are purchasing pre-prepared meals, takeaway food or eating out on a regular basis at restaurants.

Using salt sparingly is fine—it is, after all, a flavour enhancer. (Fish and chips, anyone?!) Just be aware of how much 'hidden' sodium is already in foods and check food labels when purchasing.

Salt has two main ingredients—sodium and chloride—and the sodium is what has the capacity to cause harm. Sodium is needed to help nerves and muscles function properly and to assist with fluid balance in the body. It attracts water and too much can lead to fluid retention and heart strain.

Too little sodium can cause dizziness, fatigue, headache and nausea, while an excess is linked to high blood pressure as well as heart and kidney disease.

Our bodies on average need 1000 to 1500 milligrams of sodium per day—roughly one teaspoon. Those who sweat heavily, including athletes, need more. Unless that describes you, I would consider an intake above 2500 milligrams per day as too high.

These foods are typically high in sodium:

- burgers and pizza

- certain sauces, spreads and condiments, such as soy or fish sauce

- cheese

- packaged and processed 'ready meals'

- potato crisps and salty snack foods

- processed meats and meat products, such as ham, sausages, bacon, meat pies, sausage rolls and chicken nuggets

- yeast spread (such as Vegemite).

Again, check food labels and compare products when purchasing.

For many years I have worked in the finish line medical centre at the Hawaii Ironman Triathlon World Championships. Every year, we see many athletes who have consumed too much water in an attempt to avoid dehydration in the brutal Hawaii heat. The condition this can produce is called 'hyponatraemia' (low blood sodium), which manifests as nausea, confusion, cramping and collapse. So too little salt, in some situations, can be dangerous. It is important to know your individual fluid needs on any given day and adjust for the conditions.

> **TIP**
> It is almost impossible to have a 'salt-free' diet—but adopting a 'no added salt' lifestyle most of the time is an important step in protecting your health going forward.

Good fluid intake and hydration

The body needs good hydration. We can lose up to 3 litres per day through natural sweating, evaporation, talking (who me?) and bowel fluid loss. A healthy intake of water of over 2 litres per day will keep your body hydrated and provide your cells with the ingredients they require to function at their best. Thirst is usually a sign you are already becoming dehydrated, including potential electrolyte losses (and low sodium). Don't wait until becoming thirsty to maintain your healthy hydration levels, especially if you are a heavy sweater or are active in hot, humid environments for longer than 60 minutes. However, increased salt intake during most types of daily exercise is not usually needed — consult your doctor to check if you have special needs related to your individual state of health and fitness.

Many commercially produced soft drinks and soda drinks are very high in sugar and provide 'empty calories'. Certain commercial sports supplement drinks can be of value if your exercise sessions are longer than 60 minutes, particularly in warmer weather, or if you are a heavy sweater and need to replace lost electrolytes. In most cases, good old-fashioned tap water remains your best source of hydration to complement the nutritional value of your balanced diet. In the following sections, I provide more information on the value of water, along with the benefits of other fluids, and what to watch out for.

#29 Appreciate water — understand why you need it and how much

Your body can survive without solid food for many days, but living without water is a much more difficult challenge. Your body does not store water and needs fresh supplies, usually on a daily basis. Your body is made up of between 60 and 70 per cent water, distributed throughout all body tissues, and water is essential to most bodily functions. Water is lost by various means during the day. Apart from obvious excretion from the bowel and bladder, you lose bodily fluids through perspiration, talking and breathing. (Try breathing on a bathroom mirror to see how much vapour you lose in a single breath.)

The total amount of body water you lose each day depends on your body size, occupation, exercise and other factors. In general terms, most people lose about 2.5 to 3 litres of water per day. This reduces as we age. Even when flying in a plane (and doing not much more than sitting), due to the humidity and cabin air recycle systems, you can lose up to an extra 1.5 litres of water during a single flight.

Most foods do contain some water content, but it is really through your fluid intake that you replace and maintain your body fluid needs. Because of this, it is important to understand how much fluid you need to take in each day to maintain health.

Men generally have a higher body water content than women. So it is generally advised that adult men need around 2.5 litres (around 10 metric cups) of fluid each day, while adult women need slightly less at around 2 litres (around eight cups). Younger children and adolescents require less and, as mentioned, requirements may be slightly less as you age. However, it is still important to avoid dehydration, particularly in hot weather or when exercising, regardless of age.

If you are trying to restrict your overall energy intake, fresh water is the best fluid replacement drink, but other fluids will also provide water content intake. These include milk, coffee, tea, soup, fruit juice and many carbonated soft drinks (but be wary of sugar content).

Milk is also an important health supplement and fluid replacement. (See the next section.)

Be wary of commercial drink products that pitch themselves as hydration replacements. These products can obtain high doses of sodium, potassium and other electrolytes, as well as hidden sugars.

Insufficient fluid replacement can result in various stages of dehydration, which may manifest as headaches, tiredness, dark urine, muscle weakness and perhaps some mental cognitive changes. If you are experiencing thirst, it means your body is already low on fluid, so it is best to keep ahead of the 'thirst drive'.

People who have medical conditions involving their heart or kidneys may have trouble dealing with fluid balance in the body. This may result in fluid retention, swelling or other medical conditions, so advice should be sought from your medical practitioner if you are experiencing any of these problems. On the other hand, excessive water consumption can sometimes dilute the electrolytes in the body, particularly sodium, resulting in electrolyte disturbances and a condition known as 'hyponatremia' (low blood sodium). This condition can cause headaches, confusion, dizziness and cramps.

As a medical coordinator for community events, I have seen this condition regularly in marathon and other endurance triathlon events, where individuals become too enthusiastic about their fluid replacement in the misguided belief that they will avoid dehydration if they drink excessive water. It is a fine balance between getting the right amount to meet your fluid losses and 'flooding' your system with excessive water and producing the hyponatremia symptoms. It is very much an individual thing based on your own body's behaviour and sweating ability. (See earlier in this chapter for more on monitoring your salt intake.)

The bottom line is water is important for our survival. Make sure you assess your needs based on your age, occupation and physical activity levels, and make the effort to have a water bottle handy during the day to make sure you keep your levels up. Clear urine is a good sign that your kidneys are working well, and your body is not approaching a low water or dehydration level.

#30 Enhance performance with milk

It would be a rare individual who has not tasted milk at some stage in their life. However, milk is not often thought of as a performance enhancing beverage, let alone a sport nutrition drink.

Let me state that I believe cow's milk may well be the ultimate complete health drink. It is naturally derived and is an excellent source of both macro and micronutrients. Apart from its hydrating ability, it contains important nutrients such as protein, calcium, vitamin D and multiple B vitamins, as well as minerals including sodium, potassium and magnesium. In my home, milk is known as 'vitamin M'—and that's what I tell my kids it is!

As a young child in the country, some of my earliest memories are of milk being collected from the dairy farmers' gates by transport trucks. Each morning after milking, the farmers would place the fresh unpasteurised milk in huge metal containers at the end of their farm driveways. The containers were then loaded on to the collection trucks.

When I started primary school, the state government provided every child each morning with a bottle of fresh milk, delivered in crates to the school. As I recall, the small glass milk bottles held roughly 150 millilitres each and had aluminium caps on them. They were usually left outside in the sun and the milk would often curdle.

The trick was to get to the bottles before the hot sun ruined the contents! The use of a straw was definitely optional.

In the 1980s and 1990s, we saw an explosion of marketing for various sport hydration drinks. These primarily contained water with added sugars such as glucose and various electrolyte concentrations. The power of marketing was evident when these products took hold of the sports performance market, particularly for endurance events such as distance running and triathlon, and all-day events such as cricket. However, the ingestion of these products also spilled over into general community consumption, particularly among youth and adolescents. We now often see individuals carrying one of these commercially available sports drinks and consuming them in everyday life as a simple rehydration beverage.

Because these sports drinks are often high in sugar-based compounds (glucose, dextrose, fructose), they are high in calories. They are also generally low in nutrient value when analysed for vitamins and minerals content. Cow's milk, on the other hand, contains many naturally occurring health ingredients, while also providing hydration. Milk also has the important ingredient of protein, which helps muscles recover after exercise and can even restore muscle health after vigorous occupational or manual pursuits.

If you're exercising for less than 60 minutes, you don't need to consume expensive sports hydration drinks. Water is all you need to replace the fluid and limited electrolyte losses that occur in exercise sessions of such short duration. Only when events extend beyond the 60-minute duration can fluid and electrolyte losses become more significant, and may need to be replaced during those performance periods. This can also apply to demanding manual occupations, particularly those that might occur in hot environments where sweat rates are high and energy consumption is above that of normal sedentary occupations.

NUTRITION

In comparison to most commercially available sports drinks, milk (including low-fat and skim milk) provides more energy by way of carbohydrate and healthy fat content as well as higher concentrations of naturally available sodium and potassium to deal with any electrolyte losses. It really is the ultimate hydration replacement beverage.

If you're lactose intolerant or choose not to consume cow's milk for other reasons, you will need to replace milk with an alternative hydration and recovery beverage after bouts of activity where fluid and electrolyte losses are relevant. You probably already have a preference, but note that soy milk contains about the same protein as cow's milk, and is the only plant-based milk recognised by the United States Department of Agriculture as nutritionally equivalent to cow's milk. Other options include almond and oat 'milk'—although I prefer the term almond/oat 'liquid extract'. (It must be the country boy in me coming through, but I reckon only animals produce milk. In terms of non-human production—and not ignoring the health benefits of breast milk—for me this means cows!) Again, make sure you check the sugar content of any cow's milk alternative you're considering.

It is also important to note that during high-exertion physical activities, including endurance sports performance, whole milk may not be the ideal replacement fluid due to its slow absorption through the gastric system and its higher carbohydrate and fat content, which does slow gastric emptying. Whole milk is much more suited as an after-exertion recovery drink.

However, recent studies have shown that what is known as milk 'permeate', which is the liquid product left over from the making of cheese from natural milk, does contain essential components that can be used as fluid replacement during exercise activities.

During the production of cheese, the protein and whey is kept, but the 'liquid' component is often discarded. This is the milk permeate, and it contains zero protein and zero fat but maintains the hydration ability through its water content as well as sodium and potassium ingredients. In addition, B vitamins are also retained in milk permeate, again providing it with an advantage over traditional sports drinks from the health promotion perspective. And it doesn't taste bad! It has a sweet, sometimes salty taste and cooked milky flavour.

> **TIP**
>
> If you want to consume a 'health drink' that provides you with energy, vitamins, protein and other health-promoting ingredients (and don't have a specific intolerance to it), milk is the answer.

#31 Boost your heart health with moderate coffee consumption

Recent medical evidence has shown that individuals who customarily consume between two and four cups of coffee per day have a reduced risk of death, particularly from cardiovascular disease. These finding were independent of whether the participants drank coffee with or without a sweetener added. Of course, excessive consumption of sugar is not compatible with ideal health, but in the coffee study, sugar did not make a difference at the modest amount consumed.

Studies also revealed that coffee drinkers were significantly less likely to die from any cause, including heart disease and cancer, and have reduced risk of type 2 diabetes compared with those who did not drink coffee at all. Interestingly, those individuals who used artificial sweeteners in their coffees did not live longer than individuals who drank no coffee at all. However, the researchers concluded that this may have been associated with higher rates of other negative lifestyle factors in artificial sweetener users. This included a higher incidence of obesity, inflammation and high blood pressure in the artificial sweetener user group. Another interesting note was that the benefits of coffee drinking were observed across all types of coffee consumption, whether it was ground, instant or, in some cases, decaffeinated coffee. Researchers don't yet fully understand whether it is the antioxidant effects of coffee or other component ingredients that provide the benefits.

The bottom line is that moderate consumption of coffee was associated with a longer life in recent scientific studies, whereas low or no consumption of coffee was not. Sugar may be added to coffee from a taste preference point of view, but it is important to limit this to a small amount, such as half to one teaspoon (about 4 grams). Many sweetened coffee beverages, particularly in the United States, contain far more sugar in their production (up to 15 grams). It is clearly best to avoid these sources of coffee and caffeine. The best combination? A black coffee with or without a small amount of natural (not artificial) sweetener.

While the news that the consumption of caffeine and coffee is related to longevity and healthy lifestyle is positive, there is a limit to how much should be undertaken. As just mentioned, two to four cups of coffee per day have been shown to be beneficial in most of the studies where caffeine was helpful. Increasing the number of coffees to more than five or six per day is not recommended. No evidence suggests that more is better when it comes to increasing coffee consumption.

You might wonder just exactly how much caffeine you are consuming with a cup of coffee. The answer is it varies by an amazing amount depending on how the coffee is prepared. In general, the 'average' cup of caffeinated coffee contains 80 to 100 milligrams of caffeine per serve and, overall, this is a reasonable rule to use.

However, I was recently at a conference in the United States where a presentation from University of Washington researchers looked at the range of caffeine content from over 100 coffee shops that they surveyed in the downtown Seattle area and surroundings. They purchased takeaway coffees and analysed them in their laboratory. Remarkably, they found that the caffeine content from this huge range of commercial coffee shops varied enormously — from 24 milligrams up to 240 milligrams per serve! So, you can imagine the difference in sensation you may get from almost a 10-fold difference in the caffeine content, depending on where you buy your coffee. These findings definitely explain why sometimes I find a significant difference in the flavour and buzz obtained from having my daily coffee. Fortunately, my local coffee shop is consistent. However, when you buy your coffee from a range of different locations, you can see why you might feel a different 'caffeine hit' depending on the barista, brewing time and the type of beans used. This wide variation in caffeine content can have significant consequences on the overall amount of caffeine you are consuming in a single day, particularly if you are having more than four cups in a 24-hour period (not recommended).

In addition, the same study determined that the half-life of caffeine (defined as the amount of time the caffeine lasts before being broken down in the body) varied from 2.5 hours in some individuals up to 15 hours in others. In other words, the duration of effect and benefits from consuming any amount of caffeine is also widely variable depending on your metabolism.

One interesting side point in the study was that females who are taking the oral contraceptive pill took a lot longer time to process the caffeine in their system.

NUTRITION

So, if you are a regular coffee drinker, particularly in Australia where the coffee culture is so strong, paying attention to any variations in flavour and effect from different coffee locations is important. Overall, however, you are doing yourself a favour in relation to your health practices when you attend each morning for your barista-prepared fresh coffee.

Caffeine: Harmful or healthy?

Caffeine consumption has been written about for decades. When most people think of caffeine consumption, their thoughts generally turn to coffee — one of the greatest methods of caffeine intake in the world. However, you can consume caffeine in many other ways, including in tea, caffeinated sports drinks and certain 'booster tonic' products. And some confusion continues in the many articles written about caffeine as to whether it is good or bad for you from a health perspective. No doubt for some individuals, caffeine (being a stimulant) can play havoc with cardiac conditions, causing irregular heart rhythm or unstable blood pressure. It can also cause sleep disturbance when it over-stimulates those individuals who are sensitive to it. However, at other times, caffeine is heralded as a health-promoting product.

So, what are the likely benefits? In most individuals, caffeine improves alertness and has been demonstrated to mask the signs of fatigue during activity. In addition, improved endurance and stamina have been reliably established in laboratory tests. All these features can potentially benefit an athlete at the elite level.

From a purely health perspective, concerns have also been well documented regarding rapid increases in heart rate, impairment of fine motor control and technique, and over-stimulation leading to anxiety, irritability and insomnia. Potential problems have also been associated with increases in blood pressure, mild dehydration, and the activation of heart rhythm problems in young athletes who may have had previously undetected cardiac conditions. These unwelcome side effects can occur at low dosage levels but are far more likely to occur in the high dosage range that has been publicised in sport doping reports—that is, 500 to 800 milligrams intake per day.

Every individual, athlete or not, should know his or her tolerance level and reaction to any supplement used to assist performance. I do not believe it is possible to restrict social use of caffeine due to its widespread presence in so many food products and everyday beverages such as tea, coffee and certain sports 'tonic' drinks. However, I am opposed to the use of pharmaceutical-quality caffeine in the form of concentrated tablet or powder supplementation when the intent is clearly to extract a sport performance advantage over and above that gained through natural ability and training. The benefits gained and risks associated with ingesting pure caffeine tablets are significantly different to those associated with caffeine-containing commercial beverages.

No elite athlete should experiment with pharmaceutical caffeine without medical supervision. If you are an athlete, discuss it with your doctor. Discussions should cover the indications, likely effects and risks, safety and correct dose. Moreover, I believe there is no place for caffeine supplement use in junior sports.

In everyday, non-sport use, caffeine consumption at moderate levels is associated with definite health benefits in those individuals who do not have medical contraindications to its use. However, sensitivities to caffeine consumption vary widely in individuals. Always check with your family doctor if you have any concerns.

NUTRITION

#32 Enjoy a cup of tea

The health values from drinking tea have been well established; however, the reason I am giving you this tip is not specifically related to the documented nutrition benefits.

Certainly, tea is nutritious and contains several healthy ingredients, regardless of whether the tea is caffeinated or non-caffeinated. Caffeinated tea obviously contains caffeine in varying amounts, the health benefits of which have been documented in the previous section and nearby breakout box.

In addition, teas contain minerals such as potassium, magnesium, sodium and zinc and, depending on the form of tea you take (for example, black, green, herbal or oolong), it may also contain calcium and fluoride. Tea also contains polyphenols, which are antioxidants, and these have been linked to the reduction of risk in certain diseases.

Drinking tea has been associated with a multitude of health benefits. These include improved heart health, diabetes and weight management, and perhaps the reduction of certain types of cancers. Studies around these are variable, but certainly some very positive reports have emerged.

Reports from 2022 also document lower mortality rates in regular black tea drinkers (with or without milk added). The National Institute of Health in the United Kingdom studied half a million people over 11 years. Those who drank two or more cups of tea each day had 9 per cent to 13 per cent lower risk of death from all causes than those who didn't drink tea. Yet another step towards a longer healthy life for tea drinkers.

However, the main reason I am offering this tip is for the psychological and calming benefits. As a youngster growing up in the country on our small farm, a kettle of water was always boiling on our wood combustion stove. It was a long-held tradition in the Larkins family that anyone could drop in to visit my mother and father at virtually any time of the day, especially weekends, and be offered a cup of tea made in an old Robur teapot with premium-quality tea leaves. My dad drank strong black tea (unfortunately, with sugar added) and my mother drank strong tea, with milk, no sugar. Milk first, tea second was our household rule, never the reverse! Everyone in my family, including myself, my two sisters and my brother, grew up drinking tea. In fact, coffee did not exist in our home, and I was not regularly exposed to coffee drinking until moving to university residences at the age of 17. (My first exposure to coffee was a cheap, instant, 'coffee dust' product, which I presume started life as real coffee beans at some stage!)

The point of my story is this: my mother always felt that a good cup of tea was a way of sitting down to assist somebody who was undergoing a form of life crisis or stress. My mother, Cecilia, was a great listener and many times people would visit our house to discuss their problems and seek a calming conversation with my mother over a cup of tea. To me, my mother's cup of tea was her most famous 'mother's medicine', available to all. It served many therapeutic purposes for dozens of family, friends and relatives over many decades. It helped to relax, calm and reduce stress in those who had the opportunity to share a chat over a famous Larkins cuppa. In those days, it was still common to have supper after the evening meal, prior to retiring to bed. In this way, the cup of tea at supper became almost a sedative. (Although, as discussed, caffeine can have a negative impact on sleep in certain individuals. Fortunately for me, it has never had that effect.)

Additional studies on tea have shown a variety of other benefits, including boosting your immune system and fighting inflammation. Certain types of herbal teas—such as green, turmeric and peppermint teas — may also assist with inflammation, irritable bowel syndrome, migraines and joint osteoarthritis.

It's time to put the kettle on!

> ## *TIP*
> Next time you have a friend or colleague who is undergoing stress in their life, invite them around for a cup of tea and a calming chat. That's Cecilia's tea therapy! It can help people clarify their problems and lead to their overall progression to wellness.

#33 Watch your alcohol consumption

Alcohol in moderation is not a bad thing, although I accept that many individuals do not drink alcohol and never have throughout their life. It is simply a personal choice. The types of alcohol that are available are extremely variable, from the ubiquitous beer through to the various wines (still, fortified and sparkling), as well as the multitude of spirits (the most common being vodka, rum, whiskey and gin).

Clearly alcohol is a very socially accepted part of society, particularly around mealtimes and celebratory events. It's also big business, with Statista estimating global revenue from the alcoholic drinks market for 2023 to be US\$1.6 trillion (or AU\$2.55 trillion). The responsible, controlled use of alcohol will always be with us, and I discuss the potential health benefits of wine, particularly red wine, in chapter 10. But are other types of alcohol considered health promoting? While experts may disagree with the degree of risk, sadly most concur that no amount of alcohol should be considered a health booster.

Indeed, consumption of alcohol beyond moderate amounts has definite negative effects, particularly related to aggressive or anti-social behaviour. You're no doubt familiar with the dangers that this behaviour can create.

Frequent use of alcohol may also increase the risk of high blood pressure, stroke and heart disease, cancer, liver disease, depression, fertility problems and injury. In addition, many of the tragedies occurring on our roads are related to alcohol consumption and drunk driving.

My advice here is straightforward. If you enjoy alcohol, drink responsibly and reserve it for social occasions with friends. One to three drinks per session is not excessive but you have to know your individual tolerance and limits.

Your diet and you

No single, ideal diet exists. This is evidenced by the multitude of commercially popularised diets, including the paleo diet, keto diet, Atkins diet, Zone diet, low-carb diet, ultra-low-fat diet, the CSIRO Total Wellbeing Diet ... (I need to stop listing diets here to avoid adding too many pages to this section!) And, of course, confusion persists regarding the various percentage contributions of carbohydrate, protein and fats in a healthy eating plan. The simple fact is this: there is an ideal diet for every individual. And sometimes it takes a period of experimentation (trial and error) to determine what suits your body type and metabolism best.

All of the well-known diets have their pros and cons. But, in essence, the concept of eating healthy, unprocessed foods with a good representation of vegetables and fruit, together with lean protein and some carbohydrate and healthy fats is hard to beat. It is also so much simpler for you to follow this uncomplicated plan.

Extreme swings in diet have been shown to create negative neurobiological feedback to the brain. You may perhaps achieve some short-term weight loss (through deprivation), but then often experience subsequent appetite increases and rebound weight gain that leaves you at an even greater weight than your initial starting weight.

In the following sections, I outline some easy and clear ways to sustain a consistent healthy eating plan. I do include the famous Mediterranean diet as a well-studied, proven healthy diet that is accessible and well suited to most individuals.

#34 Aim for a healthy, sustainable weight

The Australian population has a problem of excessive weight — this is well acknowledged and documented. Multiple studies show that around 67 per cent of males and 55 per cent of females in Australia are either overweight or obese. This figure has been progressively increasing in recent years.

Of more concern is that Australians aged 17 or younger are also significantly overweight, with 25 per cent of this group experiencing weight problems. By 2025, it is predicted that more than 30 per cent of Australia's youth will be overweight or obese.

Why is this happening? The answer is simple — we eat too much junk food in Australia. The standard Aussie diet now contains way too much takeaway and fast-food meals. Australians are eating fewer home-cooked meals than ever and the gold standard 'meat and three veg' meal is a rarity rather than the norm. Too many calories come from high-fat, processed convenience foods that are often lacking in sufficient nutrients, protein and vitamins. The excess calories consumed in these foods must be stored as fat and the result is easy to see — increasing numbers of people who are overweight or obese. Add to this the declining rates of physical activity participation across all age groups and it is clear why we are facing a health crisis — currently and in the years ahead.

Significant health consequences are associated with these facts. Being overweight is associated with problems of heart disease, diabetes, stroke, increased blood pressure and certain cancers. These problems creep up on you silently in the third and fourth decades of life, but the processes causing them often begin in your teenage years. It is difficult to be productive in your professional and social life if your health is below its best.

We are lucky that in Australia we have a fantastic range of natural food products covering all the important food groups. Unfortunately, too much of the modern Australian diet is based on pre-prepared foods that have been over-processed and over-refined. Fad diets such as low-carbohydrate, high-protein or high-fat diets have become quite trendy but have been shown to have no long-term effect on weight control and may, in fact, have the opposite effect. The real aim is to develop a well-balanced healthy diet to support body and brain health and function.

#35 Take some tips from the Mediterranean diet

The Mediterranean diet has been the subject of publicity for many years. While no absolute fixed definition exists as to what it involves, the general understanding of the Mediterranean diet is that it is rich in fruits, vegetables, healthy grains and heart-healthy fats. It is not only based on good nutrition principles, but also can be extremely flavoursome and delicious.

The classic Mediterranean diet is based on the traditions of the people who lived along the coastline of the Mediterranean Sea, including those in Italy, Greece, Spain and France. The Mediterranean diet encourages the consumption of naturally grown foods such as vegetables, legumes, nuts and seeds, and heart-healthy fats, particularly extra virgin olive oil. It does not contain processed foods or foods with additives such as sugar or preservatives. Many health studies have noted that people from these regions generally live a healthier life and have a lower risk of many of the standard chronic societal health conditions, such as heart disease, diabetes and stroke.

The Mediterranean diet is particularly famous for its potential benefits related to heart disease and blood vessel disorders. Experts have even suggested that the Mediterranean diet can slow or reverse the negative effects of poor nutrition and lifestyle choices in those who may be already experiencing these disorders. It can assist in the reduction of blood pressure and lipid levels, including cholesterol, as well as reduce the risk of diabetes. It has a positive effect on blood sugar control as well as insulin function, reducing the risk of low insulin sensitivity or insulin resistance. This diet packs a lot of punch!

Further studies have also suggested that the Mediterranean diet can assist in mental health and improve cognitive performance, with a reduction in the risk of dementia or Alzheimer's disease. In combination with the outdoor activities and social interactions that are common in these Mediterranean countries, it is easy to understand why improvements in memory, attention and cognitive performance all are consistently seen in people in these regions who consume some version of a healthy Mediterranean diet.

A 2022 study by Dr Jessica Bayes at the University of Technology Sydney even showed that in young male adults diagnosed with moderate to severe depression, a 12-week exposure to the Mediterranean diet had a significant improvement in their depression symptoms score.

So what foods should you be eating? The common food types associated with a healthy Mediterranean diet include the following:

- vegetables — tomatoes, capsicum, spinach, onion, carrots, cucumbers, zucchini, sweet potatoes, cauliflower

- fruits — apples, bananas, oranges, strawberries, grapes, figs, melons, peaches

- nuts and seeds — almonds, macadamia nuts, cashews, sunflower seeds, pumpkin seeds, hazelnuts

- legumes — lentils, beans, peas, chickpeas

- fish and seafood — salmon, sardines, tuna, oysters, crab, mussels

- poultry — chicken and duck

- eggs — generally chicken eggs, but occasionally also other sources such as duck or quail

- wholegrains — rye, barley, corn, whole wheat pasta and breads, brown rice, oats

- dairy — cheese, yoghurt, cow's milk

- herbs, spices and aromatics — garlic, mint, basil, rosemary, parsley, pepper, cinnamon, sage

- healthy fats — especially extra virgin olive oil, whole olives, avocado.

The classic Mediterranean diet avoids added sugars, preservatives and refined oils such canola or cotton seed oil, and certainly does not rely on convenient fast-foods that we often see in our takeaway society. The avoidance of trans fats, which are found in fried foods and margarine, is also typical of a healthy Mediterranean diet.

Interestingly, while water is the healthiest fluid that should be taken, the Mediterranean diet also features moderate amounts of red wine (one to two glasses per day). (See chapter 10 for more on the medicinal value of red wine.) Coffee and tea are also regular beverages in these regions, but soft drinks, soda or fruit juices high in sugar are not generally consumed.

You can see from the range of foods consumed that the Mediterranean diet can be easily incorporated into modern healthy living, particularly in those countries such as Australia where fresh produce is generally abundant and available. You have enormous variety to choose from. While it is not necessary to include all the various food groups mentioned here in every meal, it is generally possible to follow the principles of the Mediterranean diet on most days of the week, even if you are not a particular fan of one food type (such as seafood), or are focused on a plant-based diet.

> ## *TIP*
> By committing one or two days per week to following a Mediterranean diet plan in your life or household, you will quickly see how delicious and nutritious this type of diet is — and I predict it won't be too long before you are incorporating it into more than just one or two days per week.

#36 Pursue your (nutrition) rainbow
....

We are blessed in Australia to have an incredible range of healthy, naturally produced foods. One of the simplest ways to make sure you are eating a well-balanced variety of foods is to follow the 'rainbow principle'. By choosing foods in a range of colours each day and each week, you will expose yourself to an excellent selection of healthy foods.

Some examples of the rainbow foods to pursue include:

- green — salads, broccoli, beans, spinach

- red — tomatoes, capsicums, chilies, strawberries, raspberries, apples

- yellow — squash, pumpkin, banana, mangoes

- white — cauliflower, beans, mushrooms

- blue — blueberries, blackberries

- orange — carrot, sweet potato, oranges

- purple — eggplant, grapes, beetroot.

Protein can also be part of the rainbow selection — for example, red for lean meats, including beef and lamb, and white for multiple fish varieties and tofu.

I am sure you can add your own colours to the list and come up with a more exhaustive variety of foods. The point is simply to choose from a good selection of colours and avoid having the 'beige plate' that is so common where nutrition practices are not well followed.

Choosing a range of natural foods, and avoiding excessive processed and pre-packaged foods is the way to go. Indulging frequently in lots of fried foods or carbohydrate-laden processed foods will also result in placing our body's systems under stress — not only your heart, but also other organs such as the stomach, liver, kidneys and digestive system overall.

Counting calories

For as long as I can remember, the principles of giving advice about weight loss have often included the concept of counting calories. Most dietitians, nutritionists and weight loss programs traditionally referred to the need to reduce calories in the diet in order to lose weight. While the principle of this seems quite logical, calorie counting is not always the most critical thing in determining how to change your nutrition plan.

The number of calories required to provide the appropriate energy for your daily living is, of course, dependent on the nature of the activities, your occupation, and any sport that you may be undertaking. The basic requirement for 'normal' living is generally considered to be around 1500 to 1800 calories per day. Top sports competitors, particularly those who are participating in high-energy-demand endurance sports, will often consume 7000 to 8000 calories per day to meet their outgoing energy requirements.

The principle of balancing 'energy in' and 'energy out' to maintain weight is also a relatively logical and simple concept. If you consume more food (calories) than you expend as energy, your body will deposit the additional calories, most commonly in the form of stored body fat. This is a basic survival principle that has been around since humans evolved. On the other hand, if you are expending more energy than you are consuming, you will be in a negative energy balance and, therefore, will be burning up the stored calories in order to provide the metabolic energy required. Inevitably, in these circumstances you will most likely lose weight. However, it's not always that simple — read on!

Various weight loss programs recommend restricted calorie diets, sometimes as low as 800 calories per day. This is an extremely small amount of food to sustain for healthy living and will often lead to other unwanted metabolic effects such as ketosis. This is where the body is using ketones from stored fat instead of glucose for energy, and over extended periods can be associated with headache, nausea, brain fog and fatigue — along with generally making people quite grumpy as they go through the hunger pangs.

At the other end of the scale (pardon the pun), many foods are surprisingly rich in calories. For example, a regular latte coffee contains around 150 calories, an average chocolate snack bar contains 250 calories and even a single chocolate chip cookie can contain up to 200 calories. It is easy to see how you can exceed an intake of 2500 calories per day simply by eating three 'standard' meals per day along with a few additional snacks — especially if the snacks contain high-density, sugar-laden carbohydrates rather than healthy fruit or nuts.

One other thing that may surprise you is the amount of exercise that needs to be undertaken in order to 'spend' the calories you have consumed. Simply walking at a moderate pace expends around 500 calories per hour. If you add some slow running, you can expend up to 800 calories per hour. A stationary bike expends around 500 to 600 calories per hour, whereas swimming can be as low as 400 to 500 calories per

(continued)

hour. Obviously, the intensity and technique of the activity that you are undertaking can determine whether you expend more calories as the difficulty of the exercise goes up. The point here is that it does take quite a lot of exercise to expend even 500 calories of food consumed. After you've completed a satisfying exercise workout, if you then consume a carbohydrate-loaded soft drink and a packet of potato chips, you can easily add another 400 to 500 calories to your daily intake within a minute or two!

A better alternative to counting calories is to really look at the quality and type of food that you are consuming over the course of your daily eating program. Avoiding the heavily processed foods and sticking with healthy fruits, vegetables and lean protein will ensure that you gain good nutrition content, but do not load up with non-nutritious calories. By avoiding snacking between meals, you will also avoid the excess calorie intake. Timing your meals according to hunger and making healthy choices is more important than becoming obsessed with weighing food or counting specific calories. This is not to say that you should not become aware of—and try to avoid—the calorie-dense foods that may have a short-term satisfying effect in terms of your hunger, but do not provide good nutritious content for overall body metabolic health.

So, avoid being obsessive with calorie counting and instead implement a healthy eating plan with good energy expenditure through some form of consistent and regular daily exercise. You will then be on the path to maintaining an optimal and healthy body weight. If your goal is weight loss, then aim for a consistent exercise plan with regular expenditure of the consumed calories. You will ultimately go into a negative calorie balance, which will lead to weight loss without the need for restrictive and difficult—and usually unsustainable—dietary practices.

#37 Benefit from fasting and timed eating

You may have noticed a renewed media interest in the concept of fasting as a way of achieving health benefits. While fasting can be undertaken by many different methods, more recent evidence has emerged showing the concept of what I have termed 'timed eating' to be quite beneficial for metabolic health.

By 'timed eating', I am referring to confining your total food calorie intake to certain periods of the day, often preceded by an extended period of limited or no food intake (or the 'fasting phase'). For example, if you consume your evening meal by 8 pm on a given day and then elect to forego a breakfast meal and also delay lunch until 1 or 2 pm the following day, effectively you have achieved a fasting period of 17 or 18 hours. You can then take this a little further by only consuming a light lunch in the early afternoon and reserving your main food intake for the evening meal, again at around 7 or 8 pm. This still allows you to obtain sufficient calories for adequate nutrition, but gives you an extended period of time when the body is more stable with respect to glucose fluctuations. This is my concept of timed eating.

Traditional eating methods in modern times involve the 'three meals per day' pattern, where food is consumed initially in the morning (breakfast) resulting in a glucose spike (and consequent insulin surge), and this is then repeated at each of the two other main meals throughout the 24-hour period. In other words, large glucose spikes occur followed by subsequent insulin responses. If you add to this mix a morning tea or afternoon tea snack, particularly snacks containing highly processed carbohydrates (doughnut anyone?), you get additional glucose surges in the mid-morning and mid-afternoon, with resultant insulin responses also. Effectively, with this style of eating you are continuously providing glucose hits to your body with surges during the day, meaning the risk of constant carbohydrate overload is perpetuated.

By limiting food consumption in the early morning or middle part of the day, the high glucose surges are avoided, and insulin stress is also avoided. This allows the body to draw upon its reserves, including stored fat as a source of energy, assisting with weight loss if this is something you are trying to be achieve. This healthier pattern of timed eating also provides a metabolic 'rest period' for the gut microbiome digestive process.

I am not suggesting that you should avoid consuming anything at all during the 17- to 18-hour 'fasting' period. Fluid intake, including water, healthy juices or tea/coffee, is permitted. The avoidance of high-sugar, high-GI carbohydrate type foods is what assists with this timed eating program.

You also don't have to follow this schedule every day. One option within the concept of timed eating is to only do so on certain days of the week—your food intake is then normal on other days. One example of this is the 5:2 diet, where your calorie intake is significantly limited (600 to 800 calories) or your eating timed on two days of the week but then you have a healthy and normal food intake on the five other days.

Another method is to practise episodes of timed eating. For example, you could follow the timed eating principles of 16 hours fasting (certain fluids allowed), and then have eight hours during which you can eat healthy meals. You could follow this plan for perhaps two or three weeks out of each month, but then have a week or two weeks of more traditional times for food intake. Sometimes you need to experiment with the system that works best for yourself and individualise to your own needs. For example, if your occupational or athletic pursuits are more strenuous and/or you have high demands on your energy system during the morning (such as through high-intensity training), avoiding food intake until the early afternoon may not suit you. Nutrition is such an essential component in high-performance sport, including for recovery after strenuous training, that competitive individuals need to work out the best type of meal timing that suits their training needs.

#38 Snack
.... well

We all crave a snack at times. Sometimes, this craving is an instinctive thing between meals; at other times, it's genuine hunger that drives us to top up our food intake. It's common and quite natural.

One of the most important health practices you can adopt is to make sure any snacks you consume between meals are at least healthy. Far too often in our society, our cravings for a mid-morning or mid-afternoon snack result in the consumption of highly refined processed carbohydrates, such as biscuits, doughnuts, cakes, or other forms of sweet treats that give a quick sugar hit (because they have a high glycaemic index) but result in the dreaded insulin surge and subsequent 'crashing' effect of blood sugar fluctuations. The immediate effect of these types of snacks might be satisfying, but it is short term and hunger can return quickly, resulting in over-consumption of unhealthy, sugar-ridden, calorie-rich junk snacks.

TIP

If you need to snack, choose healthy options such as nuts, berries, low-fat Greek yoghurt, bananas or apples. In this way, you will still satisfy your craving for something to eat and will get a healthy blood glucose boost, but also will be ingesting food that provides slow release energy and delivers nutrients for your body's healthy functions. Your body will thank you.

#39 Reduce your inflammation

Most people would understand that inflammation is a bad thing. The physical external signs of inflammation are generally well recognised — even as far back as the ancient Romans. In the 1st century CE, Roman medical writer Aulus Cornelius Celsus noted the four traditional hallmarks:

1. swelling (*tumor* in Latin)

2. redness (*rubor*)

3. heat (*calor*)

4. pain (*dolor*).

Inflammation of a joint or on a skin surface is generally obvious and easily visible to those experiencing the inflammation as well as other observers. These conditions include rheumatoid arthritis (affecting the joints) and psoriasis (skin). However, many hidden sources of inflammation in the body can also have a negative impact on your health status. Less visible conditions include irritable bowel syndrome, Crohn's disease, asthma, fibromyalgia, and a large variety of other 'internal' inflammation conditions.

While the primary location of inflammation may be a specific target organ — for example, the gut — if you experience an inflammation tendency, you are also at risk of other diseases related to your inflammatory disposition. This can include heart disease, diabetes, obesity, migraine, poor digestion, mood disorders and some cancers.

Some forms of inflammation are inherited and related to your genetic profile; however, lifestyle factors and choices can also amplify and promote inflammation in your body. Fatigue, stress, lack of sleep, certain foods and other emotional stresses can amplify inflammation and cause flare ups in what may have been a previously well-controlled condition (such as irritable bowel syndrome).

Not all inflammation is bad. Inflammation is one of the body's natural defence mechanisms whereby, following some form of insult or trauma, the body sends healing and repair cells to the area via the bloodstream. In other words, a certain amount of inflammation is beneficial in an acute situation to help repair damage. Low-grade, chronic background inflammation, however, is cause for concern. In fact, the recently adopted term 'inflammaging' has been coined to reflect the long-term damage that background inflammation can have on your body, leading to more rapid aging of your entire system.

A number of foods are associated with increased background inflammation. These include high-fat foods such as fatty meats, as well as excessively refined carbohydrates such as sugar and white processed flour.

Specific foods that are known to promote chronic inflammation or activate dormant inflammation include:

- artificial colourings and sweeteners

- artificial trans fats — including processed margarines, soybean oil and most deep-fried food

- excessive alcohol

- high glycaemic index carbohydrates

- sugar and high fructose corn syrup

- vegetable and seed oils containing high omega-6 fatty acids.

NUTRITION

In contrast, some of the foods that help fight inflammation include:

- berries — strawberries, blueberries

- citrus fruits

- cold-water fatty fish containing omega-3 oils — salmon, tuna

- green leafy vegetables

- nuts

- olive oil

- tomatoes.

My message here is that chronic background inflammation is a significant health risk and is associated with increased risk of death, particularly from cardiac disease. Natural foods that are not refined or overly processed, and don't contain hidden preservatives, are the healthy choices. By keeping your body as healthy as possible and identifying your 'inflammation triggers' — such as stress, poor sleep or diet — you can avoid provoking or activating any background inflammation conditions. Again, this will help you not only live longer, but happier too.

#40 Consider supplements — maybe

The use of supplements to promote or provide a health benefit is a multibillion-dollar global industry. Many individuals are searching for the 'magic' ingredients they hope will provide them with a healthier lifestyle — whether that be through increased energy, exercise improvement or an improved sense of wellbeing generally in their everyday life. Unfortunately, many supplements used by the general public have no validated scientific support and really are an example of the triumph of marketing over legitimate evidence.

Let's take this back to basics. According to the Oxford dictionary, the definition of a supplement is 'something that is added to remedy a deficiency'. Unfortunately, this is rarely the scenario in which most supplements are consumed in our modern Western societies.

You might consider buying or consuming a supplement for many reasons, but in general these can be categorised into the following:

- to improve health

- to correct a known deficiency

- to improve performance — in life and exercise

- to build muscle (size and strength)

- to reduce body fat.

You may also be influenced by others who are taking a supplement and who provide anecdotal testimony as to what it may be doing to assist them (otherwise known as 'influencers').

Many different supplements are also available, but some common examples include:

- amino acids

- antioxidants

- calcium

- creatine

- fish oil

- glucosamine

- herbal teas

- iron

- multivitamins

- prebiotics and probiotics

- protein

- vitamin D.

Without doubt, the best source of nutrients in your diet is natural food. Your body recognises (and therefore absorbs) nutrients better if they are from an unprocessed natural food source such as vegetables, fruit and grain products. Any foods that have been over-processed, over-refined or overcooked to within an inch of their useful life are of far less nutritional value.

The bottom line is simple — if you eat a broad enough selection and variety of the key essential food groups mentioned throughout this chapter, you do not need any expensive bottled supplements.

If, however, your lifestyle includes too much processed or mass-produced food, including takeaway food options, then you might consider a broad-based multivitamin supplement containing iron, vitamin B and anti-oxidant (vitamins A, C and E) components. (This might particularly be true if you live in student housing or share a house where the overall cooking skills leave a bit to be desired! Believe me, I once lived that life for several years and know what it's like and the nutrition challenges it presents!) If you follow a plant-based diet, you also might choose a complete multivitamin that covers all the bases, or might opt for a specific vitamin supplement with nutrients that can be missing on a vegan diet, such as omega-3 fatty acids, specific vitamins, calcium, iron and zinc. Check with your GP about the supplements that might be best for you.

Other factors influencing the use of supplements will obviously vary depending on your health status, age and other medical factors. In general, my advice is that supplements should only be used when the contents are known and preferably with the input of a qualified dietitian or medical practitioner. For example, during pregnancy, women may experience low iron levels and increased demand for folic acid—in these cases, supplementation has been shown to improve the health of the mother and developing child.

In terms of evidence for performance improvement, particularly in the exercise area, very few supplements have been scientifically validated. Standout products that have been shown to be of benefit include:

- beta alanine (amino acids)

- carbohydrate

- caffeine

- creatine

- nitrate

- sodium bicarbonate.

However, these products are very specific to athletic performance and have not been validated as 'performance enhancers' in everyday life and function.

The importance of the 'placebo' benefit of supplements should never be underestimated. By definition, a placebo effect is a response resulting in improved performance after taking a product that really does not contain any significant active ingredient or nutrient. Some benefit may occur because the individual has a belief that the product will give them some improvement. In other words, the expected gains from using the product result in a positive benefit, despite the fact that the product itself may be inert or inactive when it comes to improvements in metabolic functions. The 'power of placebo' is an important component in life as well as sport performance. In fact, it is often used in providing health benefits in the traditional medical world.

One of the other critical risks with supplement use is that many products contain contaminated or other ingredients not listed on the packaging. This can result in an adverse reaction occurring when someone is allergic to or has an unknown sensitivity to an ingredient. This particularly applies with overseas products bought on the internet. These have been shown on many occasions to contain contaminants, preservatives, colourings or indeed additives including stimulants or anabolic agents that are designed to provide the 'tonic' effect, even though they are not listed as an official ingredient in the advertised product. Products bought from overseas countries that do not regulate sales or advertising of online supplements need to be used with extreme caution. This is a particular danger for athletes who are subject to doping codes, where an athlete may record a positive doping test from consuming a product inadvertently. It is a sad but preventable tragedy when an athlete's career is ruined as a result of not understanding what is in the 'magic protein powder' or other heavily promoted supplement they have purchased. All athletes are advised to seek clarification from the experienced medical practitioner connected with their sport before consuming these products.

In the normal non-athlete world, a supplement may also interfere with medication you are taking or cause a significant adverse reaction due to unknown ingredients. Again, the best nutrients, vitamins and minerals you can consume come from healthy natural foods — not from a commercial pill, powder or capsule.

#41 Understand food labelling

Although not compulsory in every country in the world, nutrition labelling for foods in Australian supermarkets is commonplace. In Australia, all packaged foods must comply with the Australia New Zealand Food Standards Code, which came into effect in 2000.

Food labelling must outline the ingredients included in the product and provide the nutrition information panel, which allows you to be informed of the contents, nutrition value and any additives that may be present in packaged foods when contemplating a purchase. Foods such as vegetables, fruit, fish, eggs and certain dietary supplements are generally exempt from labelling requirements.

I am always impressed when I am in my local supermarket and I observe customers reading food labels. I presume these people are educated in relation to their purchasing habits and are studying the labelling to look for information such as sugar and fat content and the presence of any preservatives or colourings. This allows for a healthier choice.

When studying food labelling, look for products that have low fat and low sugar content (4 to 6 per cent). Try to identify preservative or colourings or any strange names you don't recognise — this generally indicates that the components are not natural foods.

Throughout this book I emphasise the value of natural food intake. Processed foods increase the potential for adverse reactions, including the promotion of inflammatory chemicals in the body (pro-inflammatories), because so many contain excessive salt, sugar, flavourings, colourings or other fillers.

Just remember 'natural is best' and limit your processed or packaged foods to those rare occasions when the situation dictates the need for their convenience — always consume in moderation.

Nutrition labels generally must also display the amount of energy (calories or kilojoules) as well as their overall fat content together with carbohydrates, sugar, protein and salt. Generally, these amounts are expressed in grams per 100 grams or 100 millilitres of the food. This allows a percentage figure to be calculated — for example, 6 grams of carbohydrate per 100 grams of the food product represents a 6 per cent carbohydrate content. You can then compare this against another product you're considering.

Try to educate yourself, at least in the basics of healthy food labelling. I hope to see you soon in the local food shops studying the labels!

#42 Masticate more — and slowly

No, I'm not getting R-rated here! Mastication describes the action of chewing our food, and is an important part of the digestive process. Chewing your food slowly and carefully (masticating) ensures that you will derive the optimum nutrition and absorption from the foods you eat.

The process of food digestion in fact starts one step before food even enters your mouth. The mere sight of food can activate the salivary glands, which then prepares the digestive system for its optimal performance. (Hence the oft-used term 'mouth-watering' food!) Once you begin chewing, the salivary glands in your mouth increase their production to begin the digestive process. If you eat too quickly and swallow your food without chewing carefully, you are missing one of the most important steps in the digestive process. Of course, the enzymes in the lower gastric system, including the stomach and colon (bowel), will ultimately complete the digestive process, but if you don't masticate properly, you will miss a critical stage.

Saliva contains many important enzymes, including amylase and lipase. Amylase plays an important role in breaking down starches (complex carbohydrates) into sugars your body can more easily absorb and utilise. Lipase plays a different role in breaking down fats so they can be more efficiently absorbed in the digestive tract and utilised for the body's needs. In addition, if you do not chew slowly, you are missing out on two other important stages in the healthy digestive process.

Firstly, a multitude of taste buds within the oral cavity are associated with the enjoyment of food. The tongue is richly supplied with taste buds to provide the pleasurable sensation of favourite food flavours. Surely one of the great pleasures of eating is enjoying the taste? If you swallow foods too quickly, you bypass this phase.

Secondly, a feedback pathway in the oral cavity communicates directly with your brain to provide a sense of satisfaction from eating food. This is extremely important in the eating process and may also help suppress the need to eat excessively as the hunger centre in the brain registers this pathway information and may assist in helping you to avoid overeating, which will be important in your weight management process. In certain parts of Japan, where women and men live extremely long and healthy lives, the custom is to stop eating when 80 per cent full. In this way overeating is avoided and the brain has time to register the satisfaction of the food already consumed. (See chapter 10 for more on the parts of world where people live longer than average lives, known as 'blue zones'.)

So when your mother (or father) was telling you to eat your food and chew slowly at a young age, she (or he) was not only looking after your eating etiquette, but also helping you to get good nutrition practices.

My message is clear: you need to masticate often and slowly. In this way, you will ensure that your nutrition is optimised, and you will be providing your body with the best fuel to not only provide energy, but also keep all of your organs and systems functioning in their most healthy state. In this way, you can help avoid the likelihood of many illnesses associated with poor nutrition.

Yet another step in your pathway to a long healthy life.

8
Habits

In this chapter, I discuss some of my tips to improving health habits and behaviours in everyday life. Throughout this book, I stress that your own personal behaviour choices combine to be the biggest determinant of your longevity and productive healthy living. So here I discuss some of the important areas to address and optimise on your journey to a healthy 100 and beyond—and some simple everyday actions to get you there.

Look after yourself with everyday simple actions

Small, simple changes you make to your everyday habits can have a big impact over the long term. These changes can be as simple as getting enough sleep each night, and ensuring you get a good dose of 'happy hormones', such as dopamine and oxytocin. I provide some tips and actions in the following sections to help you on your way—and again, as with most aspects discussed throughout this book, starting with healthy food and daily exercise lays a strong foundation.

The actions included here combine with good nutrition and exercise to improve your overall health and longevity, and reduce your risk of heart disease, diabetes and some cancers. Again, changes can start with small efforts — for example, working on your sleep habits before you go to bed, relaxing your breathing or making sure you put on sunscreen whenever you're out in the sun. You'll start feeling the benefits of these small changes straightaway, and they only build over time.

Again, you don't have to adopt all of these tips at once. Pick a few that resonate, incorporate them into your life and keep practising them until they become a habit. Then you can look at adding something else. The aim is to slowly build your regimen of health behaviours into your week so that you build your resistance to the common lifestyle illnesses that inhibit consistent productivity and performance in everyday life. With every action added, you'll be making progress towards your healthy 100.

#43 Make sure you get enough sleep

Sleeping is an everyday function to which most people give little thought — although, if you're not getting enough, you probably give it a lot of thought indeed. When you consider that the current average life expectancy in Australia is over 80 years and that many individuals spend one third of their 24-hour day sleeping or in bed, the staggering fact is that you could spend over 27 years asleep or in bed during your lifetime. So getting the quality of that sleep period optimised certainly makes sense. (And that is also the reason you should invest in a comfortable mattress and bed!)

Sleeping might be a normal daily activity, but good-quality sleep isn't always achieved. Sleep is an essential part of your body's recovery from its normal day-to-day activities and taxing metabolic processes. Without good sleep, your stress levels rise and your functional performance declines. Long-term sleep deprivation has been associated with ill health and premature death. When looking at the lifestyle factors you need to get right, high-quality sleep is very high on my list.

While the quantity of sleep required may vary in individuals, it is really the way in which you sleep and the time spent in the important recovery deep phases of sleep that you need to get right. Deep-phase sleep represents only a percentage of your sleeping time, but is critical in obtaining high-quality and restorative sleep benefits.

In this and the following few sections, I address why you sleep, and the strategies you need to adopt to ensure that you are obtaining your best sleep quality for your needs and lifestyle. Without quality sleep, your health will be negatively impacted and that target of 100 years and beyond of quality healthspan will be harder to achieve.

Why you need to sleep

Most experts agree the reason we sleep is to repair and restore our bodies in preparation for the next day's efforts. During sleep, the body consumes less energy and quality sleep is a chance for the restorative phases of our metabolism and hormone cycles to become active. It is also likely that the brain learns new processes and creates memories during this restorative sleep phase.

Getting the optimal amount of sleep

The amount of sleep people actually get varies. Studies from the National Sleep Foundation in the United States, for example, show that the average person sleeps 6.7 hours during working days and up to 7.4 hours on weekends. In comparison, studies on elite

HABITS

athletes show that these athletes often spend eight to nine hours sleeping due to their high physical training commitments. Studies on primary school children (ages nine to 11) and adolescents (ages 12 to 15) concluded that preteens need to sleep an average of 9.25 hours whereas older adolescents also need nine to 10 hours to avoid daytime drowsiness and impaired learning performance.

For most adults, the optimal amount of sleep is around seven to nine hours. This is obviously a broad range, but sleeping for fewer than seven hours each night probably has a negative impact on overall health in the majority of individuals. (I once knew a surgeon who claimed he never slept more than four hours per night. One must wonder about whether he was functioning effectively in his overall life, let alone when in the operating theatre!)

Many people do not sleep well or get their optimal amount of sleep. Certainly some of the most frequently prescribed medications in family practice are those that assist with sleep function, including sedative sleeping tablets. However, other strategies can be put into place to get beneficial sleep. First, work out the amount of sleep that is best for you, aiming for at least seven hours. Next, you can look to ensure that your sleep environment is optimal to get restful sleep without the need for pharmacological support—which I cover in the next action.

Phases of sleep

Sleep experts describe five distinct phases of sleep:

+ *Phase 1:* This is very brief, often lasting less than 10 minutes, and is the first stage of the sleep process.

+ *Phase 2:* This phase is quite substantial, and experts estimate that you likely spend up to 45 per cent of your sleep time in phase two.

+ *Phase 3:* This is the phase when you transition between lighter sleep and into the deeper more restorative phase.

+ *Phase 4:* This is the 'deep sleep' phase, when your brain is active with delta waves.

+ *Phase 5:* This is the deepest phase of sleep, when your brain is active but your body is in a deeply immobile state. This is the only rapid eye movement (REM) stage. (The other phases are all known as 'non-REM' phases.) REM sleep is important to improve mood, memories and learning.

During phases 3 and 4, your brain undergoes slow wave sleep, and it is during these stages that restorative hormones such as growth hormone are most effectively released. Growth hormone is one the most important restorative hormones. It aids tissue repair and recovery and usually has a surge into the bloodstream at around 11.30 pm to midnight. If you do not fall asleep before this time, you can miss out on this important release of growth hormone.

In a typical sleep cycle, you move through these phases at various times through the night, with multiple periods in the REM phase when memory and learnings are enhanced. The more sleep cycles you undergo during a night, the more likely you are to go in and out of REM sleep.

HABITS

#44 Focus on your sleep hygiene

Sleep experts emphasise the importance of creating a regular routine around your sleep–wake cycle. The concept is referred to as good 'sleep hygiene' and the important factors to aim for in sleep hygiene include:

- going to bed and waking up at the same time each day

- creating a quiet sleep environment

- avoiding screen stimulation such as using mobile phones or tablets immediately before retiring

- avoiding caffeine or alcohol late at night

- avoiding heavy meals immediately prior to retiring (not going to bed on a full stomach)

- the use of quiet, relaxing music or sounds (I like waves or rain sounds)

- using meditation, slow breathing or a mindfulness session to promote rapid sleep onset

- sleeping in a cool environment rather than high heat or humidity.

> ## TIP
> If you find yourself lying awake with your brain busy or ruminating over life issues (and who hasn't done that?), it is better to get up rather than lie restlessly in bed. Sometimes some non-stressful reading can assist. You can also try the

old-fashioned tactic of a glass of warm milk, which is now backed up by science. (Milk contains tryptophan, used by the body to make melatonin, which regulates the sleep–wake cycle, and serotonin, which regulates appetite, sleep, mood and pain.

#45 Watch out for sleep deficit and sleep deprivation

Experiencing regular days of insufficient sleep below optimal levels is often referred to as being in 'sleep deficit'. When the lack of sleep becomes extreme, it is known as 'sleep deprivation'.

Regular bouts of insufficient sleep lead to increased levels of stress hormones released from your adrenal gland and upregulates your natural glucocorticoid response — including increased levels of the main stress hormone, cortisol. This can cause lethargy, fatigue and premature aging of your cells.

While chronic sleep deficit or deprivation have an overall cumulative effect on your health and life performance, studies in elite athletes have shown that poor sleep for one single night before an event does not have much impact on performance. Studies looking at endurance performance, leg strength and fatigue associated with oxygen demands have shown that athletes can perform very well despite not having a great night's sleep the night before an event. This lack of sleep is often due to time zone changes or anxiety related to an upcoming important performance the next day — and perhaps you've experienced something similar before a big presentation or important meeting. However, two consecutive nights of sleep deprivation can certainly result in below par performance.

HABITS

#46 Monitor your sleep
....

No doubt you intuitively know whether you have enjoyed 'a good night's sleep'. You can also take advantage of the multitude of wearable devices available that track your sleep, providing data on quality, time and wakefulness. Apart from maintaining good sleep hygiene (covered in action 44), certain supplements have been shown to be associated with improved sleep quality and potential reduction in night-time cramps. These include melatonin (the naturally occurring sleep hormone from the pituitary gland) and magnesium. (Melatonin is available without prescription for people over 55.)

#47 Avoid sleep disorders
....

The experience of 'not sleeping well' is something every one of us has had at some stage, even if only for one night. However, several well-recognised sleep disorders can mean the experience is much longer than one night. I cover some of these disorders, and how to avoid them, here.

Insomnia

Insomnia is defined as having difficulty getting to sleep, waking frequently or waking too early. It can occur as a brief incident during some acute life stress situations and resolve just as quickly. However, it can become a chronic condition for some people.

Most Australians experience insomnia at some point in their lives, and about one in 10 people have at least mild insomnia at any given time. It is more common in women and elderly people.

The most common symptoms of insomnia are:

- having difficulty falling asleep

- waking a lot during the night

- waking up too early and being unable to go back to sleep

- not feeling refreshed on waking.

The two broad types and causes of insomnia are as follows:

1. *Primary* insomnia occurs when no underlying cause is found, and the condition becomes chronic. This is very common.

2. *Secondary* insomnia occurs when an underlying cause is present, such as anxiety, depression, stress or other general health disorder.

Treatment should be directed at the primary cause if one is identified. However, general treatment principles also need to address:

- improving sleep routine and hygiene (refer to action 44)

- managing stress

- introducing relaxation and meditation techniques

- treating the medical condition

- using medication (occasionally, and for short-term use only)

Sleep apnoea

Sleep apnoea, also known as obstructive sleep apnoea, occurs when a person's throat is partly or completely blocked while they are asleep, causing them to stop breathing.

HABITS

During apnoea, breathing can stop for just a few moments or for up to 90 seconds. These episodes can happen many times a night. An apnoea sufferer is often unaware of these episodes but will wake feeling tired. Sleep apnoea ranges from mild to severe. In severe cases, sleep can be interrupted hundreds of times each night.

Sleep apnoea can affect anyone but is more common in people who are middle aged or older, who snore, who are above their healthy weight or who have a family history of sleep apnoea.

The symptoms of sleep apnoea include:

- pauses in breathing while sleeping, which may be noticed by other people

- snoring

- tossing and turning

- waking up gasping or choking

- feeling tired and unrefreshed after sleep.

Individuals who experience sleep apnoea are also more prone to other medical conditions, such as

- diabetes

- stroke

- poor memory and lack of concentration

- headaches

- moodiness, depression and personality change

- lack of interest in sex, and impotence in men (often a pretty good motivation for men to get this sorted out!).

If you have mild sleep apnoea, sleeping on your side, losing some weight and avoiding excessive alcohol during the evening may be all that is needed to treat the problem. Other strategies include stopping smoking or using nasal decongestants (if acute local obstruction is present).

For moderate to severe sleep apnoea, more active treatment may be required, including:

- a fitted night splint or mouthguard to assist airway flow

- a continuous positive airway pressure (CPAP) machine, which feeds pressurised air into a face mask to hold your throat open while you sleep — frequently used for more severe sleep apnoea.

Snoring

I know this is a topic that resonates with many of my friends (no names mentioned to protect the guilty). You likely know someone who snores — and you can become all too familiar with the condition if that person lives in the same house as you! And I'm not talking just about men here — I have a female friend who told me about her own snoring. (Although she referred to it as 'snurring' — 'much more feminine', she told me!)

People commonly snore due to the following:

- late night alcohol

- smoking

- being overweight or obese

- a cold, sinus or allergy problems

- sleep position, especially sleeping on the back

- breathing through the mouth.

Identifying and addressing any of the factors just listed is a good place to start to combat snoring. For example, losing weight, avoiding late night alcohol and changing sleeping position are all proven helpful methods — some of which have other flow-on health benefits. If sleep apnoea is also occurring, a CPAP machine (see preceding section) can assist.

If your child snores because they have enlarged tonsils, this can affect their overall sleep quality, and your doctor may ultimately suggest surgery to remove their adenoids and tonsils if other strategies don't help.

'Restless legs'

The feeling of 'restless legs' is a condition of the nervous system where you have an urge to move your legs to relieve unpleasant sensations, such as burning, tingling, aching, itching or a feeling of something crawling under your skin. Involuntary uncontrolled jerking movements of the legs may also occur at night.

The cause of these feelings is not well understood, but certain health problems can lead to restless legs syndrome. These include chronic kidney disease, iron deficiency anaemia, diabetes, arthritis and Parkinson's disease.

Conventional treatment for restless legs syndrome is relatively non-specific and success varies. Things to try include hot baths, heat packs and leg massages, reducing caffeine and alcohol intake, stopping smoking, managing stress and introducing good sleep hygiene.

Remember—healthy sleep is critical for body recovery and repair. It allows your body to deal with the demands of everyday pressures and stress. Poor-quality sleep will have a cumulative impact on your quality of life and ability to live to your 'healthy 100 and beyond' goal.

#48 Dream sweetly

Dreaming is something that has always fascinated me. I don't know anyone who hasn't experienced dreaming at some stage, and studies suggest that everyone dreams.

Dreams can be quite random and sometimes you can experience a recurring dream. Sometimes they make sense and other times they are completely nonsensical. They can be enjoyable, fun or downright scary. Dreams can occur in black and white images, but most people experience colour in their dreams at some stage.

Dreams can involve other people whom we know, but frequently complete strangers appear. A particularly important event during the day might trigger a dream of a similar content that night. A dream, for example, might involve an individual, a topic or an object that you encountered during the previous day. At times, a dream can be so vivid that you even become aware that you are not awake and recognise you are in a dream phase. (Reaching this point in a dream likely results in you waking up before the content of the dream is completed.)

Sometimes you can remember your dreams very clearly the next day, while others may disappear completely from your memory. This is because not all parts of your brain are active when you are sleeping so the memories of the dream are not always being recorded. Indeed, some studies have shown that 95 per cent of the content of a dream can be lost within 30 minutes of a person waking up.

TIP

If you want to remember the content of a dream, write down as much as you can remember within five minutes of waking up—before your brain loses the memory.

Dreams most frequently occur in the phase of deep sleep that involves rapid eye movement (REM). Typically, an individual can move in and out of REM sleep on multiple occasions each night. Although dreaming occurs during deep sleep, this is not always the most restful phase of sleep. During dreaming in the REM phase, the prefrontal brain cortex usually shuts down, resulting in disinhibited brain activity. This is why some dreams can have bizarre, nonsensical content. Other parts of the brain, known as the hippocampus and amygdala, become very active during dreaming.

The purpose of dreaming is not well understood. Dreaming normally reflects activities in our subconscious mind, but theories related to its purpose — and what our dreams might mean — have been studied by philosophers and psychotherapists since before the times of Sigmund Freud. Dreams can sometimes involve reliving a problem in our daily life so that a solution is achieved during the dream. Artists and songwriters have been known to create masterpieces during dream phases.

Nightmares are generally disturbing and frightening dreams associated with an unpleasant experience. They are usually triggered by a negative experience or reflect mental health concerns, psychiatric problems or life stresses, such as occupational, financial or relationship issues. Recurring themes in your dreams tend to reflect unresolved or even unconscious issues in your life, and seeking therapy can help you not only stop the dreams but also—and more importantly—address these underlying issues.

> ### TIP
> Do you have a recurring dream, pleasant or otherwise? Does the theme make sense to you based on previous life experiences? If you identify a negative recurring theme, seeking psychological therapy could help you deal with the dream process and eradicate it from your life.

HABITS

It is fair summary to say that dreams have been studied by many experts for decades (if not centuries). The true nature of why we dream, and the explanation of the contents of our dreams, has eluded definitive answers in many cases. Interpretation of dreams is quite subjective by outside individuals and may mean more to the individual experiencing the dream than the therapist interpreting it externally.

Importantly, the quality of your sleep and dreaming experience determines much of your energy and wellbeing the following day. Trying to have good sleep hygiene practices, avoiding stressful activities in the hour prior to sleeping and learning meditative processes can all assist in avoiding negative dream experiences.

As someone who has been a prolific dreamer over my lifetime, I wish I had all the answers for you, but understanding dreams is an ongoing challenge for the neuropsychiatric world. What I can give you is a simple hope your dreams are all good, sweet dreams.

#49 Get your daily DOSE
of happy hormones

Getting a good night's sleep isn't the only thing that will improve your mood during the day. You no doubt know how much more enjoyable your day is when you are in a 'good mood'. Of course, many factors create the environment to put you in a good mood, but generally your mood is controlled by a series of chemical processes in the body particularly related to brain neurotransmitters. Indeed, a particular group of hormones is known as the 'happy hormones'—which I have dubbed the 'DOSE' hormones. These are a group of hormones that contribute to your wellbeing and mental health status being quite positive. Getting your daily 'dose' is one of my most important messages in this book to assist with enjoying a happy and productive long life.

My four DOSE hormones are:

- **d**opamine

- **o**xytocin

- **s**erotonin

- **e**ndorphins.

Each of these specific hormones has a role to play in your health status and mental wellbeing, and you can promote their activity in many ways.

Dopamine

Dopamine is a neurotransmitter manufactured in the brain that acts as a messenger between your nervous system in the brain and the rest of your body. It is the primary hormone in the 'reward centre' in your brain, with roles in many important bodily activities such as memory, motivation, mood, attention and sleep.

Dopamine belongs to a group of chemicals known as catecholamines, of which adrenaline (epinephrine) is probably the one you will be most familiar with.

While dopamine has many roles in the body, its primary actions are associated with pleasurable reward and motivation, memory, attention, behaviour and cognition, as well as arousal and sleep. In this way, it enhances mood and improves cognitive function in your day-to-day behaviour. When you are doing something that you enjoy, your brain recognises this and produces more dopamine, which then improves the pleasure of the activity and encourages you to seek more of that rewarding feeling. This reward response is also unfortunately why certain unhealthy foods and junk foods containing sugar are so addictive. They also contribute to dopamine release, and while this is not the desired result, it explains why junk food can be so addictive and lead to unhealthy eating patterns.

High dopamine levels can also give you a sense of euphoria, make you feel energised and contribute to an increased sex drive. People with low dopamine levels often feel unmotivated, unhappy, and fatigued. They experience mood swings and have trouble sleeping.

You can increase your dopamine via natural methods, and one of the simplest is to regularly exercise — a potent dopamine enhancer. Other pastimes such as meditation, yoga and activities that make you feel happy or relaxed also increase dopamine production in the brain. Foods that are high in magnesium and the amino acid known as tyrosine also serve as building blocks for dopamine production. This means some important foods for enhancing dopamine include fish, chicken, dairy products, avocado, green vegetables, tomatoes, wheat germ, nuts, apples and chocolate (great news for the sweet tooths out there!).

HABITS

Certain drugs mimic the natural neurotransmitter effect of dopamine, and these are often used to treat medical conditions such as Parkinson's disease, depression and low sex drive. In certain medical conditions such as schizophrenia, bipolar depression and other psychotic conditions, dopamine function can be abnormally high. In these cases, the prescribed medications are designed to block dopamine receptors.

My dopamine message is clear — by participating in regular physical activity and exercise as well as eating healthy foods, you will increase natural production of dopamine, which will enhance your mental state and contribute to your overall wellbeing.

Oxytocin

Oxytocin is one of the pleasure hormones in the body and is known as the 'love hormone'. It is produced in the hypothalamus of the brain and released by the pituitary gland.

One of the most important functions of oxytocin is to assist women during childbirth by stimulating muscle contraction of the uterus to help with the labour and delivery. Following childbirth, it assists with the mother's milk production and the emotional bonding process between the mother and child. On occasion, it can be administered artificially to induce labour or assist with the labour process.

Oxytocin can also be naturally released during other activities, including exercise and sex. In fact, the reason it has been termed the 'love hormone' is because it is associated with the pleasurable feelings of connection accompanying and following orgasm during sexual activity. (In this context, I suspect many people might choose this activity ahead of exercise to get their pleasurable oxytocin hit!) Studies have also shown oxytocin is released during other forms of physical contact, such as massage, cuddling or hugging, and is even associated with pleasurable music.

You can see why it is important to obtain your daily dose of oxytocin as part of your overall health program. I will leave it to you to decide which activity you select to facilitate the oxytocin release!

Serotonin

Serotonin is a neurotransmitter also known as 5-hydroxytryptamine (5-HT) that enhances the way your brain communicates with other nerve cells in the body. Serotonin is mostly found in the gut (90 per cent), but also in the brain itself (10 per cent).

Serotonin is associated with improved happiness and memory and also has a role in hunger and sleep quality. A lack of serotonin can lead to depression, anxiety and other mental disorders.

Serotonin plays a major role in mood and is often known as the 'feel good' hormone. It contributes to your sense of calmness, emotional stability and happiness. It also plays a role in aiding digestion by helping expel toxic products from the gut. Having a healthy gut microbiome helps optimise serotonin levels in your body. (Refer to chapter 7 for more on gut health and improving your gut microbiome.) Serotonin also plays a role in other important body functions, including wound healing, bone health and sexual desire.

You can improve your serotonin levels in a number of ways, and one of the most important is — you guessed it — exercise and physical activity! Foods containing tryptophan, an essential amino acid, also help you increase your serotonin. These foods include salmon, turkey, eggs, cheese, nuts and oats.

HABITS

Serotonin is really the hormone I consider an 'all round performer' that can enhance your health and lead to a happier, longer life.

Endorphins

Endorphins are also important hormones in your body. They are opiate-like substances, with their chemical structure similar to pethidine, morphine and other medically used drugs. As such, they can assist with pain management and help improve your emotional mood, even to the point of potentially providing a mild euphoric effect.

People who exercise regularly often describe an 'exercise high' associated with the natural release of endorphins that can occur during consistent physical activity. (This is also known as the 'runner's high' in people who are regular runners. I have been a consistent runner for many years but, unfortunately, I am still pursuing the day when I reach the ultimate runner's high! That is not to say I have not had many exercise sessions where I have felt a great sense of achievement and emotional reward from my exercise sessions. Perhaps I have experienced an endorphin high without realising it at the time!)

Other pleasurable activities such as receiving a massage, eating pleasurable food and even sexual activity can increase endorphin levels. At the other end of the spectrum, endorphins are also known to be released when the body is experiencing pain or stress. As an example of this, I remember hearing stories as a youngster of military personnel who had been badly wounded during a battle but did not realise until much later. The natural endorphins being produced during the stress of the activity managed to provide them with natural pain relief.

Your body releases many types of endorphins during triggering activities, but the beta endorphins are the primary endorphins involved in stress relief and pain management. Some of the beta endorphins have even been reported to have a stronger effect than the well-known opiate drug morphine. The endorphins released during exercise can assist with mood elevation and treatment of depression, stress and anxiety. The feeling of improved self-esteem that comes from completing an exercise task or challenge is also associated with the endorphin release.

Reduced endorphins in the body can be associated with poor sleep, mood disorders and general body aches and pains including fibromyalgia. Endorphins work together with dopamine to enhance your enjoyment of activities including exercise. As such, they are complimentary (synergistic) hormones that can help you increase overall gains and benefits.

In addition to exercise, you can promote endorphin production and release in your body through eating dark chocolate, meditating, laughing or engaging in other pleasurable activities such as watching a favourite movie or TV show. You'll no doubt agree — it should not be too hard to include these activities in your week to obtain your endorphin surge!

Overall, you can see how important it is to get your daily DOSE of happy hormones. They can all work in harmony to provide you with a healthier and happier mindset and provide many physical benefits. The wellbeing effects are self-evident. By incorporating exercise and healthy eating into your day, you can ensure that your DOSE will be achieved, and you will be on the pathway to a healthy, productive 100 years and beyond.

Have you worked on getting your DOSE today?

HABITS

#50 Breathe
.... **easy**

Including a section on the importance of breathing may seem a bit strange. I am reasonably confident that over the last five minutes, whatever you were doing before reading this, thoughts of breathing were not high on your list. Breathing is one of those automatic functions that is critical to your existence, but often does not get much attention paid to it.

Those who practice meditation or yoga will attest to the importance of breathing techniques and regular breathing exercises in producing a greater sense of calm and relaxation. Psychologists always recommend breathing exercises for those suffering from panic and anxiety as a way of reducing their stress in a difficult situation. Athletes who are preparing for a competitive performance will often practise slow breathing techniques to focus their mind and get themselves into a more relaxed state prior to an event. And if you've ever suffered from nervousness in an exam, presentation or other situation, you likely know that some form of relaxed breathing can be of assistance when the techniques are properly learned.

Some studies have shown that when you're about to perform a difficult task, focusing on a positive outcome and reducing distractions is beneficial. When you are concentrating on slow breathing techniques, your brain can shut out other distractions such as stress or auditory stimuli that may distract you from the task. It is almost as if the brain directs its focus to your breathing efforts and then blocks out all other stimuli, including stressful thoughts.

Athletes often use deep, slow and focused breathing before a significant moment in their performance — such as before launching into a high dive from a diving tower, running up for a high jump performance, or taking a shot on goal in a football game. I even remember watching an international darts competition (did someone say 'athlete'?) where the competitor was attempting to shoot an important score but performed focused, slow breathing with his eyes closed prior to launching the dart missile. (Fortunately, he opened his eyes prior to the launch!)

The physiological role of breathing in delivering oxygen from the air to your lung pathways and ultimately into your bloodstream for energy is probably pretty obvious. This system is controlled by your autonomic breathing system and, as stated, likely does not get much thought or attention as you go about your daily activities. Yet breathing is one of the most important functions of your life and works together with your heart (providing its pumping action) to deliver oxygenated blood around your body.

Meditation teachers emphasise the importance of focusing on one simple activity such as breathing to get into a proper meditative state. This can often be as simple as concentrating on slowly breathing in and slowly breathing out while relaxing the various muscles in the body to achieve a calm, relaxed state. Many apps or instructional videos also offer other slow breathing techniques in various forms. You can determine which options works best for you, but a combination of timed inhalation, a period of breath holding, then timed exhalation is generally the right combination for most people. My personal favourite is the 3-3-3 method: inhale slowly over 3 seconds through the nose (this communicates directly with your brain centres), hold and relax for 3 seconds, then exhale through your mouth over 3 seconds.

By learning good breathing techniques and using them when needed, you can reduce your stress and anxiety and contribute to your overall sense of calm and wellbeing. Over the long term, this can lower blood pressure and improve heart health, again contributing to a longer, healthier life.

HABITS

#51 Quit smoking — right now!

Historical studies suggest the use of tobacco began around the 1st century BCE when the people of Central America discovered tobacco leaves and used them for smoking, usually in religious and sacred ceremonies. Subsequently, tobacco use spread through North and South America where it was popularised by the indigenous peoples.

As global seafaring travel evolved, Europeans were gradually exposed to these smoking habits. After Christopher Columbus's voyages and once Portuguese and Spanish sailors (among others) began visiting these countries, the popularity of tobacco use blossomed. Interestingly, in early times tobacco was also used to cure certain illnesses such as asthma, bowel problems, fever, burns, earaches and sore eyes. As recently as the 1960s, cigarettes were being marketed in the United States and other locations, and even endorsed by medical practitioners, as a way of promoting and *improving* lung function and treating asthma. How our knowledge has changed!

Since the 1970s, the publicity regarding the negative effects of smoking has been widespread. Studies have clearly identified the links between smoking and throat and lung cancer and other respiratory diseases starting in the mouth, throat and spreading down to the lower airways. However, the adverse effects of smoking are far more widespread and include negative impacts on heart disease, stroke, diabetes and other cancers, including bowel and prostate.

Smokers also have a slower healing potential, which has a significant impact on their recovery from surgery. Postoperative infection risk is also higher in smokers. This is related to the microvascular damage caused by smoking, and this has an impact on healing and infection resistance throughout the entire body.

Tobacco contains 2550 known compounds, and tobacco smoke itself contains more than 4000 compounds. In tobacco, the primary hazardous compounds include at least 43 cancer-producing compounds such as nicotine and nitrosamines. Tobacco smoke can also contain carbon monoxide, herbicide, fungicide and pesticide residue, together with tars and many other substances that impair your body's defence mechanisms and result in immunosuppression. In this way, smoking virtually affects every cell type in your body.

According to the Australian Institute of Health and Welfare (AIHW), tobacco is the leading cause of preventable disease and injury in Australia. The AIHW also highlights that tobacco use is the leading cause of cancer in Australia, contributing to 44 per cent of the total cancer burden. In developing countries, smoking has been associated with over 85 per cent of all cancer deaths in men, and 90 to 95 per cent of all lung cancer deaths have an association with smoking.

I cannot think of one better example of poor lifestyle choices where men and women both suffer from the condition I have termed LRD: 'listener receptor deficit'. The dangers of smoking and the impact it can have on overall health are so well known, and yet individuals who smoke continue to ignore the available information. These people not only need to be counselled for their smoking behaviour, but also treated for their LRD!

While knowledge has expanded and advertising that promotes smoking has been reduced, the tobacco industry continues to search for innovative ways to encourage smoking. For a significant period of time, sport was seen as a perfect outlet for smoking promotion. Fortunately, smoking advertising has now been banned (although promotion of alcohol and betting continues to be an issue).

Legislation has also been introduced to prevent smoking in aircrafts, restaurants and other public places in most parts of the world.

HABITS

However, if you've visited Europe recently, you will have seen that smoking is still very commonplace in countries such as Greece. The message is clearly not getting through to the extent that it needs to be.

Statistics from the AIHW suggest that around 11 per cent of Australians over 14 years of age were smoking in 2019. The trend has been declining significantly over the past 20 years. The expenditure on all tobacco products has also dropped dramatically over recent decades—from $44 billion in 1990 to $17.2 billion in 2018. The highest consumption of tobacco is in the 45 to 54 years age group, but regular consumption has been documented in children as young as 14 years of age.

In 2022, it was estimated from ABS data that around 12.6 per cent of males and 8.2 per cent of women were daily smokers. Unfortunately, the use of e-cigarettes (or 'vapes') has increased in recent years, with two in five current smokers using them in their lifetime. People who use vapes now make up almost 9 per cent of the population. Experts also believe increased rates of vaping are also linked to increased smoking rates in young people. (Refer to chapter 3 for more on this.)

On the plus side, 23 per cent of Australians claim that they are 'ex-smokers', while 63 per cent report that they have never smoked. While these are encouraging figures, reducing the current use of tobacco products in the community remains a challenge.

Exposure to second-hand smoke is also not without its risks. It has been linked to increased risk of cardiovascular disease, lung cancer and many childhood respiratory illnesses, including sudden infant death syndrome (SIDS).

The health risks of smoking are indisputable. It does not seem logical to voluntarily expose your body to a major illness cause.

My message is clear — you need to quit smoking right now, and avoid any exposure to it. You will then be able to add to your recipe for a longer, healthier life.

For help with quitting smoking from health professionals, access your local Quitline service — go to www.quit.org.au or ring the helpline on 13 7848.

#52 Protect your skin — health is more than skin deep

Data from the AIHW highlights that skin melanoma is the third most common cancer in Australia after breast and prostate. Fortunately, however, melanoma is dropping out of the top 10 causes of death in Australia. The number of deaths for 2022 was estimated to be around 1315, with roughly twice as many males dying as females. This represents 2.7 per cent of all cancer deaths. The reduction in the overall number of deaths is a result of more frequent early detection and better treatment options becoming available, particularly with the advances in immunotherapy for cancer treatment.

Experts still estimate that 16878 new cases of melanoma were diagnosed in 2022. This represents 11.2 per cent of all new cancers diagnosed.

With advancements in treatment options, the five-year survival rate for a melanoma diagnosis is now around 92 per cent, again according to AIHW data. Nevertheless, over 60000 Australians are still currently living with a diagnosis of melanoma. That's a lot of stress to live with.

HABITS

Prevention of melanoma is absolutely critical, and adequate protection from harmful UV rays when outdoors is my main health message in this area. Always wear sunscreen and use UV–protective long-sleeved clothing and hats when outdoors, either in an occupational or a recreational situation. Australia has one of the highest incidences of skin cancers in the world, and federal and state governments have been very active with skin health protection messages. The 1980s campaign promoting 'Slip, Slop, Slap' (slip on protective clothing, slop on sunscreen and slap on a hat) has been important in teaching all individuals, particularly from a very young age, the importance of protecting the skin when outdoors and exposed to harmful UV rays. This campaign has since been expanded to include 'Seek' and 'Slide'—seek shade and slide on sunglasses—highlighting the importance of avoiding the sun where possible, especially between the hours of 10 am and 3 pm, and protecting your eyes from sun damage.

> ## TIP
> Get any unusual skin lesion investigated and once you're over the age of 40, book in for a regular skin mole check. An experienced skin cancer professional can assess a skin lesion that has changed in size or colour or has bleeding tendencies.

If required, a skin biopsy can also determine what type of skin cancer you may have. While melanoma is certainly the most publicised skin cancer, many others are also possible, including basal cell carcinomas, squamous cell carcinomas and other less common types of skin cancers. All need to be treated, usually by surgical removal.

Your skin is one of the most important (and largest) organs in your body—so look after it. By minimising your risk of this common cause of health problems and possible death, you are increasing your options for a long, healthy life (and healthspan).

Use it, train it, nourish it—or lose it

You have likely heard the phrase 'use it or lose it' many times in your life. My variation here can be applied to many components of your body but, in this instance, I am specifically referring to your muscles (particularly skeletal muscles), your heart (which is cardiac muscle) and your brain. You need to treat all of them as you would any functioning organ, body part or structure that needs to be kept at its optimal health. Our bodies respond well to the application of controlled challenges and stress.

Skeletal muscles provide you with your dynamic mobility, stability and balance around major joints, and your overall shape. They provide power and locomotion. Muscles decline in strength by 1 per cent per year from the age of 30 (or 10 per cent per decade). However, training a muscle with regular activity—using a mixture of aerobic and resistance or strength work—helps slow the aging related changes of muscle decline. In many circumstances, this decline can be reversed by regular exercise.

Remember—your heart is also a muscle and needs to be used and trained, even with low- to moderate-intensity challenges, in order to maintain its optimum performance and stop the decline of a weak floppy heart.

Finally, the brain (while not technically being muscular tissue) responds to repeated challenges and has been shown to have less chance of developing senile changes such as memory loss, cognitive decline and dementia if you keep using it for day-to-day simple challenges.

Hence my advice to 'use it, train it, nourish it—or lose it'. Introducing activities to maintain these three important systems in your body is such a simple concept, and I provide many such activities in the following sections. Follow the actions and tips outlined here and you are a long way towards progressing on the path of a healthy, long lifespan.

#53 Get moving every day — incidental activity

While most exercise guidelines are prescriptive in describing the number of sessions per week or the number of minutes per day that are required to achieve health and fitness benefits (and I include some of these guidelines in chapter 6), it is also important to consider the impact of your incidental activity.

Incidental activity relates to those periods during the day when you move about in the course of completing everyday duties. This activity might occur in the workplace, in the home or in other locations that are not part of your normal structured exercise program. A good example is parking your car (or getting off your tram or bus) a little further from your end destination to increase the time that you spend walking. If you work above the ground floor in an office or other building, another example would be walking up and down the stairs rather than taking the lift. Both of these options (which I cover in more detail later in this chapter) provide you with some additional exercise in the process of going about your usual day's activities.

Similarly, although you may have a favourite coffee shop at the base of your building, there is probably one that serves equally good coffee five minutes down the street. By walking to that other coffee shop and back, rather than using the nearest one in your building exclusively, you have added an additional 10 minutes' walk to your daily activity program.

Once you start looking, you can find ways to increase your incidental exercise in most situations. When next you are at an airport, for example, observe that the escalators are often located adjacent to a set of steps. Here is a perfect opportunity to walk up or down the steps rather than using the escalators (particularly if going down). Of course, if you're carrying heavy or difficult luggage, you are forgiven for using the escalator or lift! (I'll admit I've been guilty of using the travelator myself at times when running late to get to the plane departure gate — but I'm usually running on it if you do see me!)

My message is (again) simple. You often have opportunities during the day when you can stand and move around a little more, rather than follow the sedentary lifestyle that is so common in modern society — especially workplaces. Looking for little incidental activity opportunities can easily add up to many minutes of activity per day, and contribute to your cumulative target of 30 minutes minimum per day of aerobic exercise. Have a look around your workplace or home and see what opportunities you have to do some extra time on your feet — and make sure next time you visit the supermarket or Bunnings, you park as far from the entrance as possible!

HABITS

#54 Stand up for yourself

The simple act of standing up has often been taken for granted by some of us and not considered a potential source of health gains and fitness. (Of course, people with mobility issues don't take standing up for granted at all.) You may feel the concept of standing upright implies a passive activity without expending any energy. However, recent scientific studies have shown that the simple act of standing (when compared to sitting or lying) leads to the burning of energy and initiates muscle activity.

When you are standing, the muscles in your lower back, pelvis, hips and limbs are activated. This muscle action provides you with greater stability, balance and a sense of body position (known as 'proprioception'). The constant work required from your muscles to maintain the standing position also consumes energy, hence it promotes calorie consumption. It also stimulates loading of the muscles by requiring body weight and posture adjustments—especially if you focus to stand up straight, with shoulders back and down and stomach tucked in.

You've no doubt seen or heard of the recent trend in workplaces for stand-up desks, whereby office workers are encouraged to stand while working, and so avoid prolonged periods of sitting and gain more health benefits. This correlates with the study findings of the benefits of standing activities in energy consumption and muscle stimulation. Even the simple act of standing up from your desk and walking around for a minute or two during the course of a busy meeting or work activity provides you with some muscle stimulation. It will also break the monotony of prolonged periods of inactivity when sitting. So do yourself a favour when you are sitting for any long period of time by changing to a standing posture and gaining important health benefits.

TIP

As an added bonus when standing, try standing on one foot and then the other for 10-second repeats. (Brushing your teeth provides a perfect opportunity for this.) Just make sure you go back to two feet on the ground if you feel unstable.

#55 Take the stairs

....

Stairs are a beneficial piece of 'exercise equipment' that are available to most people every day. When ascending or descending stairs, you are using a wide variety of core pelvic and leg muscles. This simple exercise activity provides a muscle strengthening benefit and contributes to your balance and improved stability.

Studies have shown that when climbing stairs, the number of calories consumed can be quite impressive. Values of up to 1000 calories per hour have been demonstrated in exercise studies using runners on stair climbs. The actual energy expenditure depends on the intensity and speed of the climbing and your body weight. A heavier individual, for example, at a faster pace equals more calories burned — and more benefit! An 80-kilogram person ascending stairs at a moderate walking pace can expect to burn around 500 to 600 calories per hour.

You might experience many circumstances during your day when you have to move from one floor of a building to the next. Most people in these situations will choose to use a lift or elevator, even if they are only ascending one or two levels. Unless you are carrying heavy equipment or have a particular injury, using the stairs (which are usually located adjacent to the elevator) is a simple way of adding some more incidental — and effective — exercise to your day.

By taking the stairs, you are not only expending a few more calories to assist with metabolism boosting and weight loss, but also giving your core, pelvic and lower limb muscles a workout, creating strength gains. While stair climbing and stair running races are a recognised sport in their own right, the simple act of walking up some stairs when you are next in a shopping centre, airport or your office building will also give you an exercise workout that is beneficial to your overall health program.

HABITS

I look forward to passing you on the stairs when we are next in the same building!

#56 Adjust your parking habits

No doubt at some stage during your week, you need to drive to your local supermarket, hardware store or other commercial location such as a shopping mall. Most of these locations have large car parking areas, with hundreds of car parking spaces available for customers. It is human nature to want to seek out the parking space that is closest to the entrance door of the facility you are visiting. While this might seem reasonable, logical and even practical at the time, I want to suggest that here is another opportunity for some extra exercise — simply by parking a greater distance from the entrance.

Of course, inclement weather such as a rainstorm or the need to carry very heavy items back to your car may preclude you from parking a major distance from the entrance. Nevertheless, in many other situations, you likely have the opportunity to park on the furthest side of the car park and then use one of the available shopping trolleys to transport your purchases back to your car. By doing so, you again include some additional walking steps in the normal course of your day — also contributing to your aerobic exercise commitment. Walking an extra one or two minutes each way between your parking space and the shopping facility allows you to accumulate more time towards your goal of 30 minutes of exercise per day. If you're catching public transport to the shopping centre instead of driving, you can apply a similar principle and get off one stop earlier.

Try this small change to your usual habits to give yourself that little bit of an exercise boost as well as some thinking time in the course of a busy day.

#57 Own a dog!

A dog is the best piece of exercise equipment you will ever obtain!

Many individuals spend a great deal of money on health club and gym memberships, as well as purchasing home exercise equipment such as exercise bikes, rowing machines or treadmills. I agree that all of these activities are commendable when it comes to convenient physical activity, including aerobic and strength training, but one piece of exercise equipment is frequently overlooked and may be the most beneficial one that you can own. I am talking about buying yourself a dog!

I have many patients that tell me that part of their exercise regimen is 'taking my dog for a walk'. I correct them by saying that it is not them taking the dog for a walk, but the dog taking them for a walk! The commitment and responsibility of owning a dog, particularly a larger or working-breed dog that requires extended outdoor exercise on a regular (usually daily) basis, means that you have to commit to that outdoor walking session. This simple commitment locks in a regular aerobic session. Thus, your dog is providing you with the motivation of doing an exercise session that you may not otherwise do! Your dog may well be the greatest 'personal trainer' you will ever have.

When I was growing up on a small rural farm property, our family dogs got plenty of exercise simply running around the farm all day.

HABITS

Domesticated dogs based in a family home do not usually have that same luxury. At one stage, I owned an Alaskan malamute dog named Shimagun ('Shimmer' for short). Shimmer *loved* to run! He was very energetic and suited my own personal need to get a run in several times per week. He particularly loved to run to the beach at the end of the street where I lived at the time. Getting him to the beach was easy — it was flat-out race pace on the way there. Coming back was another story, however. The trouble for me was his strength. He was never keen to return home until he was ready. He would lag behind me on the return run and pull so hard on my arm that my shoulder would ache at the end on the run session. I guess it was good strength training for me as well as the aerobic workout!

Given that you should be aiming to build up to an exercise session of a minimum of 30 minutes per day, it is a relatively simply gesture to take your dog for a walk around your local suburbs, or along a nearby beach track or parklands trail in order to reach the 30-minute goal. In this way, both you and your dog gain the benefits of a daily dose of exercise.

Many people will also vouch for the fact that owning a dog, especially a puppy, is a great way to meet people! Dogs have a way of getting you engaged in a conversation with others, not just fellow dog owners. Who knows? A dog might be a new way to expand your friendship circle. Or maybe even meet your new life partner?! Your dog enhances your social connectivity options — yet another add-on benefit for a long and healthy life. (I cover increasing your social connection in much greater detail in chapter 10.)

So next time you are considering what piece of home-based exercise equipment you may like to purchase, consider a dog as your best investment. If yours is a strong as my Shimmer, you may get a strength workout as well as the aerobic session. Certainly, your dog is highly unlikely to be gathering dust and cobwebs in the corner of your garage, which is commonly the fate associated with many unused exercise bikes and home treadmills!

Pets—a health supplement?

I'm reasonably sure I don't need to convince pet owners of the benefits pets bring to their lives. However, you may not be aware that dozens of scientific studies back up this anecdotal evidence. These studies show the physical and mental health benefits linked to having a pet as a companion.

Of course, many pet choices are available, but the most common pets are dogs, cats, rabbits, guinea pigs, birds, fish or even something more exotic such as a snake or lizard.

Certain pets, such as dogs and cats, can sense an owner's mood and emotional state and react in a way that provides reassurance and comfort when needed. This can obviously help reduce stress, anxiety, and even depression in some people. The mere physical contact with a pet, especially the furry kind, can potentially lower blood pressure and provide a sense of calm. In addition, engaging in conversation with your pet is soothing—and they rarely disagree with you!

Pets can provide unconditional love and affection and often have pretty low demands—and nothing is better than their enthusiastic greeting on arriving home at the end of the day.

I outline in the previous section the value of owning a dog in providing a regular exercise routine. The benefits of less stress

(continued)

HABITS

and more walks can transfer into better health and the need for fewer visits to your GP for certain stress-related illnesses.

Owning a pet definitely comes with certain responsibilities (including, feeding, grooming, vet visits and health care) but this can give both structure and routine to your week. Pets also provide important company, which negates the social isolation that can affect many individuals, particularly in later life. This is actually one of the key reasons pets are so important, especially for single people living alone.

Hence, the benefits of owning a pet far outweigh any responsibility that comes with that ownership.

It's time to start planning and consider which pet might suit your lifestyle. Good luck making your choice.

#58 Look after your joints — they keep you moving

You can obtain your daily dose of cardio or aerobic exercise in many ways. However, most of these options do involve weight-bearing activities such as walking, cycling, using an elliptical trainer or even running. It makes sense then that you need to look after your weight-bearing joints in the lower limbs in order to optimise your options for these exercise sessions.

Understanding joint health and the role that arthritis, particularly osteoarthritis, can play in your lifestyle is important. Looking after and protecting your joints is an essential component to making sure you are able to pursue a balanced exercise program that suits your health goals.

Arthritis affects all age groups in our community and presents in many variations, including genetically inherited, inflammatory and post-traumatic causes of joint pain; however, the most common arthritis, and the one you likely recognise, is osteoarthritis. Some known predisposing factors include joint injury, alignment issues, being overweight, genetics, infection, and other factors which can disrupt the sensitive joint surfaces or important lining tissues that nourish healthy joints.

While many predisposing factors cause the development of osteoarthritis, particularly in weight-bearing joints, the end result is primarily the loss of the protective cushioning cartilage (articular cartilage) covering the ends of the bone surfaces. This results in reduced impact protection and the breakdown of cartilage cells, which then causes joint swelling, inflammation and pain.

The impact of osteoarthritis in the community is enormous, with millions of dollars a year spent on various treatments as well as creating an economic impact through loss of productivity in the workplace. The Australian government estimates the annual burden of all arthritis costs to be around $14 billion, representing 10.3 per cent of disease burden spending.

Strategies to look after your joints and prevent injury are to stay at a healthy weight and — of course! — exercise. Exercising for 30 minutes a day, including some resistance training and gentle stretching, helps joints stay mobile and strengthens the muscles that support all joints, including your knees and hips. If you develop joint pain, have it assessed by your doctor to make sure it doesn't develop into a longer term problem. To avoid injuring your joints as you get older, focus on low-impact exercises such as walking, cycling or swimming. (Refer also to chapter 7 for some tips on foods to eat to fight inflammation.)

HABITS

Understanding the common symptoms of osteoarthritis

+ *Pain:* Pain is the primary symptom of osteoarthritis that causes most individuals to seek medical help. It may initially begin as pain related only to certain activities but, as the disease progresses, pain can be disabling in day-to-day life, impacting sleep and work, and sometimes causing pain at rest.

+ *Swelling:* Every healthy synovial joint (such as the shoulder, hip, ankle, elbow or knee) has synovial fluid. This fluid serves a number of important roles, including joint lubrication, cushioning protection and, most importantly, nutrition for the articular cartilage cells (chondrocytes). The synovial fluid is produced by the sensitive synovium (lining of the joint). When the synovium is irritated by any number of processes, excessive synovial fluid is produced. Unfortunately, this fluid is not of high quality and therefore does not provide the important functions just mentioned. When the synovial fluid contains irritant chemicals, this process can stimulate the pain receptors causing excessive joint pain as well as joint swelling (known as an 'effusion').

+ *Stiffness:* Joint stiffness may occur for several reasons. Sometimes it is related to poor-quality synovial fluid losing its lubricant ability. More commonly, stiffness is associated with loss of movement as the joint gradually changes shape with bone osteophytes (or 'spurs') occurring around the joint margins. Later, thickening of the joint capsule occurs, and ligaments lose their elasticity and prevent the joint from achieving its normal end-range movements. This can have an impact on joint function and accelerate wear processes, particularly in lower limb joints such as knees and hips.

+ *Weakness:* Joint weakness and fatigue is associated with muscle function loss around the damaged joint. As the joint becomes progressively sore, individuals will often modify the way they use the joint, resulting in muscle atrophy. This can mean the simplest tasks, such as getting out of a chair, climbing stairs or walking up a ramp, become more difficult and lead to increased pain and reduced confidence. The resultant deconditioning can cause apprehension and even instability, causing collapse or falls.

+ *Deformity/malalignment:* Malalignment issues cause uneven loading and wear on the sensitive joint surfaces producing specific increased breakdown of the articular cartilage. Sometimes the malalignment is genetic—for example, from hip dysplasia or leg length deficiency—or can be post-traumatic following injury or certain surgical procedures, particularly in the knee.

+ *Instability:* When joint malalignment reaches a certain stage the angulation of the joint may result in a person having a sense of the joint moving or giving way. This is particularly relevant in the knee where stretching of the soft tissue capsules/ligaments on one side of the joint can lead to a lack of support. This makes individuals very apprehensive with certain aspects of their functional mobility and can result in falls.

+ *Crepitus:* Crepitus refers to the various 'noises' such as creaking or crackling heard when a joint is moving or weight bearing. This is usually associated with the breakdown of the articular cartilage where uneven

HABITS

(continued)

patches result in roughening of the remaining articular cartilage. While not a concern on its own, it does reflect the evolving breakdown of the joint surface and may result in irritation of the joint, producing the inflammatory synovial effusions and swelling.

+ *Reduction in functional capacity:* This happens when the preceding symptoms progress to the point where individuals become limited in their ability to enjoy everyday activities such as walking, golf or exercise, or even simple day-to-day functions such as shopping.

#59 Get treated for osteoarthritis pain

In the ideal world, treatment programs for osteoarthritis pain aim to address all of the symptoms listed in the nearby breakout box and minimise them to the best level possible. While complete eradication of all symptoms is frequently not achievable, many strategies can be introduced to deal with the primary symptoms and allow arthritis sufferers to return to a realistic level of function.

These strategies include:

- *Patient education:* This allows the patient to understand their condition, take responsibility for many of the management strategies and set realistic expectations on what they may achieve.

- *Pain management:* A variety of simple medications such as paracetamol, topical ice or massage gels can provide simple pain relief. This will also allow some of the other therapies, including exercise programs and rehabilitation, to be undertaken more comfortably.

- *Non-steroidal anti-inflammatories:* When joint swelling and inflammation is obviously present, short-use oral anti-inflammatory agents can be used to settle the inflammation process and reduce swelling as well as assisting with pain relief. Your doctor can discuss this option with you, along with any associated risks caused by co-existing conditions.

- *Stronger medications:* The use of stronger pain relief (such as opioids), has a very limited role and serious potential side effects. Again, discuss with your doctor but, generally, if you require narcotic-based medications, other strategies need to be looked at more thoroughly.

- *Physical therapy:* Issues such as weakness, stiffness and joint swelling can be assisted by various treatments provided by a qualified physiotherapist, exercise therapist or other allied health clinician trained in the management of osteoarthritis. In addition, the therapist can plan a home exercise program to help with self-management between formal therapy visits.

- *Strength training:* A guided resistance/strength training program under the care of an experienced therapist can have dramatic benefits in improving joint pain, function and patient confidence. In addition to the formal resistance training sessions, patients can be instructed in a follow-up home exercise program that involves some strength exercises to maintain the benefit.

- *Load modification:* If any trigger factors for the joint pain have been identified (such as excessive kneeling, flexing,

HABITS

high impact or prolonged standing), ways of reducing these loads in a patient's day-to-day activities can be devised. These modifications can go a long way to allowing a patient, even with end-stage disease, to function well without the need for more aggressive interventions.

- *Weight loss:* Patients who are excessively overweight are known to experience more joint pain, particularly in the lower limbs. There are some significant research studies which show that patients who lose 10 per cent of their body weight have a reduction in their knee joint pain score of 50 per cent. This is a very significant pain management strategy and needs to be addressed early.

- *Nutraceuticals:* Many products are available that do not require medical prescription but are marketed for their joint pain benefits. Products such as glucosamine, fish oil, turmeric and other 'natural anti-inflammatories' are widely available. Many patients do report an improvement in pain and swelling with their use (although this is not yet consistently backed up by research). This industry is also not subject to the rigid regulatory guidelines demanded of mainstream pharmaceutical manufacturers. While I do not advocate spending a lot of money on unproven supplements, patients will often have a trial of these products for a three- to six-month period to see if they assist with their pain management.

- *Injection therapy:* At the simplest level, this might be an injection of corticosteroid to assist with joint inflammation and swelling and allow the joint to respond better to the other therapies. (Repeated injections of corticosteroid are rarely required.) Joint viscosupplementation (hyaluronic acid; HA) agents help restore the joint fluid to its more normal status. HA injections are synthetic derivatives mimicking ideal synovial fluid and have a high success rate in appropriate patients for restoring lubrication, limited cushioning and providing some nutrient value to the damaged articular cartilage. They can be of great assistance in joint preservation but are not known to regenerate new cartilage cells at this stage. Other injections such as stem cells (primarily derived from fatty adipose tissue or bone marrow) are extremely expensive and are still subject to research. They may have benefit in reducing pain and swelling, but any predictable benefit on articular cartilage regeneration (regrowth) has not been established.

- *Surgical options:* These are usually the last resort if the preceding treatment options are not working. Surgical options include the following:

  — *Arthroscopy:* The role of minimally invasive arthroscopic surgery in the management of medium- to end-stage osteoarthritis remains controversial. While it is true that arthroscopy cannot replace damaged joint tissue (it can only remove it), my experience has been that it has a definite role in improving those patients who have mechanical symptoms such as locking, catching or documented loose bodies, which are causing significant pain episodes, instability and joint swelling. As always, talk with your doctor about the potential usefulness of this option.

  — *Joint realignment surgery:* Knee and hip realignment procedures can be performed to deal with excessive malalignment and can assist in slowing the progression of joint deterioration and avoiding the need for more significant joint replacement surgery for many years in

HABITS

appropriate patients. These decisions need to be taken after discussion with the treating clinician.

— *Joint replacement surgery:* When all of the appropriate non-operative treatment measures have failed to provide adequate pain relief, joint replacement will be discussed. Expertise and surgical techniques continue to evolve; however, following joint replacement surgery, the expectation would be that patients obtain significant pain relief, return of function and the ability to return to many of their previous lifestyle activities. Many patients even return to very active lifestyles after joint replacements, including skiing, sailing and tennis. Again, realistic expectations need to be discussed prior to surgery.

Joint osteoarthritis is a major cause of disability and healthcare costs in the community. The causes and symptom combinations are generally well documented and many non-operative interventions can be considered. It is important to undertake optimal non-operative treatment (whether that be short term or long term) before deciding that major joint replacement surgery is required.

Given that so much of the advice in this book revolves around the importance of exercise and being physically active to enhance your health, you can see why I have emphasised looking after your joint health as a key health behaviour.

#60 Set an exercise challenge

While it is important to adopt a regular physical activity and exercise routine in your general lifestyle, it is also helpful to set some targets and challenges. By setting a challenge for yourself, you motivate yourself to aim for a specific end point. This challenge may be as simple as participating as a family in a fun run (in which you are able to walk if you choose), or could be a triathlon, hiking expedition, ocean swim, or even a regular bike ride with friends. Even elite athletes who are training at high intensity will sometimes become bored with their training program, but they always have a forthcoming challenge such as a championship, team selection or qualifying event to motivate them. In a similar way, in your everyday exercise life, setting some target for the future reminds you why you are out there following your consistent exercise pattern.

Targets and challenges do not need to be complex or difficult. It is important to also set yourself some minor small stages as targets along the way towards your end goal. Setting some achievable interim steps can help you maintain the motivation and commitment to your overall training program. Of course, motivating yourself to begin a training program can be difficult, particularly on the cold and wet mornings, but having a target in mind helps you maintain your enthusiasm for the task. A certain reward comes from achieving the small targets and this can also help you with your compliance and motivation towards the overall health goal or challenge you have set for yourself.

HABITS

TIP

Even if your goal is long term—for example, weight loss over 12 months—set some easy, staged goals to get there. Divide the end result into smaller, simple targets. You will get a buzz from reaching that set smaller goal and will more likely continue the positive path. As a bonus, you will also likely get a DOSE surge as well! (Refer to action 49, 'Get your daily DOSE of happy hormones', earlier in this chapter.)

#61 Find your preferred cardio option

On many occasions, I have been discussing the importance of aerobic and cardio activity with my patients when my background as a runner at international level gets raised by them. Usually, it will be when I'm discussing the importance of aerobic activity in providing many of the health benefits outlined throughout this book. When I try to get patients to introduce some aerobic activity into their lifestyle, they often respond with something like, 'But you are a runner, and I hate to run!'

Statements like this give me a great opportunity to explain to people that running is only one of the forms of cardio and aerobic exercise that is important. Yes, I am a runner (or at least I used to be when I considered myself an athlete), but as long as you are moving, using large muscle groups, you are getting the required aerobic and cardiac benefits. Your body can't tell the difference between walking, swimming, cycling, rowing, skipping and using an elliptical trainer. It only recognises that it is moving using large muscle groups and, therefore, you are activating the important chemical processes that are associated with health benefits.

Your heart rate increases, blood flow increases to your muscles as well as your brain, and the neurochemical turbo boost that you get from these exercise hormones is also promoted.

Although running is an efficient use of cardio time if you are able, it is not your only choice. I personally had to move away from running as my preferred aerobic activity after I had knee surgery. Learning to adapt has allowed me to continue to pursue the cardio health benefits I want you all to enjoy.

Just pick something, and move! You don't have to be a runner!

#62 Chill out with cold immersion

No doubt you've heard the phrase (or been told to) 'chill out' or 'take a chill pill'. Usually this advice is given by someone attempting to help during an experience of anxiety or other stress. It turns out this suggestion may have some scientific merit.

Are you a chilled person?

In recent times, cold-water immersion events, including bay swims, regular cold-water swimming clubs ('Icebergers') and cold immersion rooms (cryotherapy), have become increasingly popular, used regularly for their purported health benefits. Often these practices are promoted by health influencers, celebrities, bloggers and some athletes. However, scientific studies are now starting to support these rituals.

Cold-water immersion practices are in fact not new and have been practised for many decades. In Scandinavia, for example, polar ice swims and immersion in ice lakes are popular as a way of promoting health benefits. Some of these annual public participation events attract significant media coverage.

Athletes also commonly have recovery sessions after sport competitions that involve wading (or even full immersion) in cold sea water. This aims to reduce muscle soreness and assist with some types of injury recovery. Immersion in cold water causes vasoconstriction (shrinkage of the blood vessels), which then reduces the amount of bleeding, swelling and inflammation in an injured area. Another common practice at elite sporting clubs is for athletes to soak in an 'ice bath' for five to 10 minutes after vigorous competitions, especially after contact sports such as football. Cold therapy immersion rooms, where the body temperature is rapidly lowered, can also be used.

HABITS

Scientific study in this area supports the use of cold therapy, showing athletes have reduced muscle soreness and some faster recovery from injuries, particularly soft tissue injuries where bleeding and swelling is a limiting factor.

Advocates of cold immersion therapy also insist that it can improve your circulation, deepen sleep quality, improve energy, and reduce inflammation in your body. Some studies suggest that people who habitually practice cold-water immersion techniques can reduce the effects of aging and, therefore, live a more productive and longer life. (This sounds appealing and is certainly on theme for this book.) Some evidence also suggests that cold immersion therapy may stimulate your immune system, which theoretically would improve your ability to fight illness.

Few studies have looked at the effect of cold immersion therapy on mental illness. Nevertheless, people who practice this therapy will often feel a sense of invigoration and improved energy, which can only be a good thing when looking at overall wellbeing benefits. No doubt this is another way to get your 'happy hormones' dose (discussed earlier in this chapter).

I am certainly not advocating cold-water immersion therapy as something everyone can jump straight into. In fact, if you have high blood pressure or cardiac conditions, it could be quite risky. You must seek medical advice before attempting any of these cold immersion therapy techniques. For those who practice cold therapy regularly, the general consensus is that you only need a few minutes of exposure in an extremely cold environment to get health benefits. Following the exposure, you need to warm up quickly by drying off, putting on warm clothes and consuming some warm beverages or food. It is important to warm up gradually, however, because changing from a very cold environment to an extremely hot one (for example, by taking a very hot shower) can cause dramatic changes in blood flow to the heart and brain and may also be a health risk.

More research is needed on the values of cold immersion therapy, but it is undoubtedly gaining popularity in the community across many age groups, not just athletes. If you are given a medical clearance to try it out, start with small duration exposures in the beginning until you get used to the cold-water experience.

> ## *TIP*
> Research also shows that having a cold shower for between just one and three minutes can provide similar benefits to cold-water immersion therapy. So perhaps start with this if you're not sure about jumping in an ice bath or cold lake! (Again, check with your GP first.)

Working out where you are in life

In Australia, studies on illness patterns and mortality show that the area in which you live can have an influence on your longevity and healthspan. This is primarily based on access (or lack thereof) to good healthcare services and acute medical care in the unfortunate event of an injury or illness.

People in rural areas in Australia do not tend to live as long as those in the built-up metropolitan cities. This again primarily relates to access to medical care. One clear example would be in the event of an acute heart attack. The ability to have medical attention within the critical first few minutes can determine the difference between survival and death. Access to those trained in CPR and, even more importantly, access to a defibrillator in the event of a cardiac arrest have all been shown to increase survival opportunity. Hospital access is also a major factor.

In the following sections, I outline tips and actions for when you live in — or travel to — different locations. These might be as life-critical as knowing where the closest defibrillator is, or as beneficial to your health and wellbeing as minimising jet lag and spending some time beside the seaside.

#63 Understand why postcodes matter

As you no doubt know, the regions of Australia are divided into postcodes. (In the United States, these are referred to as 'zip codes'.) Postcodes are used by Australia Post to help get your mail to you, by identifying the geographical location in which you work or live.

Quite simply, the area — or postcode — in which you live can determine your access to healthcare. In a continent the size of Australia, it is impossible to have sophisticated medical care facilities available to all on short notice. We depend on our country and rural population to provide us with the farming and primary production businesses that allow our nation to function so well. Other parts of the world do not always have that opportunity. Nevertheless, your postcode can have an influence on your medical care options and might influence your choice of residential location as you head into your later years.

The good news for those in more remote locations is the continuing evolution of internet facilities and other telecommunications options that allow remote access to medical care (such as telehealth) and advice on an almost instantaneous basis. If you live in a more remote region, make sure you know the appropriate numbers for easy access to your local hospital and medical facilities in the event of an emergency.

#64 Live near a defibrillator

Defibrillators, one of the great advances in medical support, are truly life-saving devices. A defibrillator delivers an electric shock to a heart that is in cardiac arrest and has stopped beating. The carefully measured shock allows the heart to reactivate its electrical control mechanism and return to a steady heartbeat when other treatment options may fail.

You understand the importance of having first aid skills, including the ability to do CPR (cardiopulmonary resuscitation) when someone has collapsed and has no pulse. The most likely cause in this situation is going to be a cardiac event, including a cardiac arrest. Obviously, because the heart has stopped beating, blood is not circulating around the body. Most importantly, blood is not reaching the brain, and it only takes one or two minutes of oxygen deprivation to cause permanent brain damage or a fatal event.

By delivering cardiac compression, the heart may start pumping again and return to some function. However, in many situations the CPR heart compressions only provide temporary blood circulation in an emergency, with the heart not yet beating of its own accord. The ability to deliver a defibrillator shock reactivates the heart's own beating mechanism.

The window available during a cardiac arrest to try to get the heart beating properly again is very short — between one and three minutes. Having access to a defibrillator in these circumstances is critical in getting a positive outcome. In the past, defibrillators were quite expensive and often complicated to operate. In more recent years, defibrillators have become quite portable and lightweight with the cost reducing dramatically to around AU$1500 or less. Using a modern portable defibrillator is also quite easy and intuitive, with the new models having a built-in audio instruction system that activates when the defibrillator case is opened. Instructions are clear and simple, even if the user has not had experience with using a defibrillator in the past. Through private fundraising and government subsidies, defibrillators are now commonplace in most public-use spaces such as supermarkets, sporting arenas, sporting clubs, hotels, schools and even in busy shopping malls and walkways. Knowing the location of the nearest defibrillator is absolutely critical when you are working in an office building or other site where there is a chance it may be required.

Any organisations that own a defibrillator also need to regularly check that it is fully charged and operational (even though it hopefully will never need to be used).

Defibrillators are truly one of the most important pieces of first aid equipment you can have in your workplace or sporting precinct. While cardiac disease and heart attacks are still very common, this piece of equipment can ensure survival from a cardiac arrest and lead to an individual returning to a full and productive life.

#65 Minimise jet lag

You likely know the challenge of trying to travel comfortably and arrive at your destination in a healthy state — including minimising jet lag effects.

Jet lag is a topic that has been a subject of discussion for many decades. Its effects are highly individual and variable, but generally jet lag includes fatigue, reduced performance and difficulty sleeping when travelling to another time zone. Jet lag results from the disturbance of the body's natural biorhythms, which control your day–night and wake–sleep cycles. In most circumstances, individuals do not experience jet lag symptoms unless they travel through time zones that are more than three hours' difference from their home destination. Studies show that for most people flying in a west to east direction causes more body clock disruption than flying east to west.

In my experience, the number of strategies offered for prevention and treatment of jet lag seems to be almost as numerous as the number of flight destinations available to travel!

The following simple measures have stood the test of time in helping to eliminate or minimise jet lag symptoms:

- *Check your flight times:* Travelling on an overnight flight from your destination (arriving in the morning) can assist with getting more rest/sleep during the flight and help to offset the amount of fatigue at the arrival destination.

- *Arrive in daylight:* Arriving at the destination during the early or middle of the day allows you to settle into a new destination and experience some daylight. Try to remain awake until the normal sleep time of the arrival destination to adjust to the appropriate evening sleep pattern.

- *Do some exercise:* Even a simple walk around the local streets can help your body clock adjust to the new location and assist with sleep. (I find this also helps me get my bearings and learn about the new neighbourhood I'm visiting.)

- *Stay hydrated:* Remaining well hydrated on the flight helps you avoid the headaches that can be associated with fatigue and jet lag. Water should be your preferred healthy fluid, but juices and other non-alcoholic beverages all provide hydration. Limit alcohol to modest amounts.

HABITS

- *Eat healthily:* Eating light meals on the flight and not having a heavy meal prior to retiring on the first evening in the new destination can assist with time zone adjustment.

- *Use melatonin:* Melatonin is the naturally produced hormone that controls your sleep–wake cycle and is primarily produced by the pineal gland. Many studies show use of melatonin tablets can assist in adjusting to the time zone. Usually, a small dose (2 to 5 milligrams) is taken in the hour or so prior to retiring to bed at the new destination and this helps to reset the body clock to a local sleep pattern.

- *Get adequate sleep:* Sleep is restorative and energising so it is important to try to get adequate sleep in the new destination time frames to assist with fatigue and jet lag reduction.

Jet lag affects individuals in different ways and many people will have their own strategies that they have developed over the years. In any event, find what works for you — and keep in mind that it is a temporary condition. Your body will find a way to settle into its biorhythms at the new destination within a few of days after arrival.

#66 Get a dose of sunshine — but stay sun smart

While I love all the seasons and enjoy the changes throughout the year, if I was given a single choice, I would probably prefer the warmer summer months. Summer fashion, together with the ability to do activities outside and feel the warmth of the sun, is a mood lifter for me. Indeed the role of sunshine in health maintenance is well established.

Apart from the obvious ability to spend more time outdoors in warmer weather enjoying the sun, and the opportunity for outdoor activities including exercise, the extra advantage is obtaining vitamin D. Vitamin D has been shown to be an important ingredient in bone metabolism as well as assisting with general metabolic health, including reduction of inflammation. Sunlight is the best source of vitamin D, and your levels can go down over winter, especially if you live in a colder climate.

Perhaps you've also heard of the well-documented medical condition 'seasonal affective disorder syndrome' (SADS). This syndrome is associated with winter, when people spend more time indoors away from natural sunlight, and particularly with countries that experience long hours of darkness during the winter. SADS is linked with a reduction in the production of certain hormones and a loss of vitality, with increased lethargy and potentially some level of depression. Getting outdoors in the sun allows for the natural production of these hormones to be reactivated and gives your spirits a lift.

HABITS

I once worked with a well-known orthopaedic surgeon who described his own experience with the SADS over a number of years. One of the treatment strategies suggested at the time was more exposure to ultraviolet (UV) light. So this particular surgeon recommended standing in front of an x-ray viewing box (which does put out some UV light) as a means of getting exposure to the light frequency and, hence, improve mood. I did try it on one or two occasions, but rapidly lost interest after a couple of minutes because I found it extremely boring. To me, it seemed much simpler to go outside for a walk or an exercise session to get natural sunlight!

> ## TIP
>
> Be sun smart whenever you're outside and avoid excessive exposure to harmful ultraviolet rays. Wearing sun protective clothing including hats, skin and face protection is critical in avoiding skin damage, including cancers such as melanoma.

So, one of the important strategies in helping to live a long and healthy life is to spend more time safely outdoors in the sun. This could include planning holidays in warmer environments, particularly with a beach close by.

#67 Be beside the seaside — or any good view

One of the early tips I was given in life regarding living longer was that people who live near the water, or who can see water from their homes, lived a longer life. I think this advice may have been given to me by a real estate agent who was trying to sell me a house that was close to the water with fantastic views. But it did stick in my head. And I did end up buying that house, mainly due to its wonderful views of the sea. I convinced myself when I was on my deck, looking out to the bay and observing the ever unpredictable yet hypnotising emotions of the ocean in the distance, that I was living a healthier life simply because I bought the house. Perhaps not true. But nonetheless the view was amazing.

I guess the point of this is that living in an environment that is calming or conducive to your mental wellbeing is a great way to make sure you're living a contented life.

It really doesn't matter whether your favourite place is near the beach or simply in a rural area where, instead of water views, you enjoy the sound of the birds and the quietness of a rural environment, especially at dawn as the sun signals the beginning of a new day and nature bursts into life. Maybe a view of a dam will substitute for the ocean! I am fortunate to regularly visit a beautiful rural cottage, with distant ocean views and native parrots, kookaburras and galahs visiting my deck to greet me early in the mornings. Pure bliss!

Just simply having a place where you feel relaxed and can walk out the door to do some exercise in a pleasant environment will contribute to your mental health and give you a boost. Whether that place is in the bush, forest, around the lake or along a beachside area, it will encourage you and make your exercise session more pleasant.

So, if I have the choice, seeing water and being near the water is certainly my preference. This also applies to holidays, where I again prefer to be near a beach or other body of water.

But we are all individual and unique in what nurtures our emotional state — the key is for you to decide for yourself which situation gives you that dopamine-filled, happy hormone rush, and then try to spend more time in that environment to improve your overall wellbeing.

#68 Keep up to date with your vaccinations

The practice of administering vaccines to humans in order to assist with protection against illness has been around since the late 18th century, when smallpox was the major threat. Since that time, dozens of different vaccinations have been developed in each century to provide protection and immunity against severe illness or even death from various infections.

Since 2021 and the COVID-19 pandemic, the topic of vaccinations has become very prominent in the media. Of course, some individuals do not believe in vaccinations, be it for ethical, religious, medical or other reasons. Since the onset of the COVID-19 pandemic in January 2020, however, one of the major reasons for reductions in severe COVID illness and death has undoubtedly been the introduction of the various vaccines and subsequent boosters that have been available since 2021 and through to 2024.

The concept of vaccination is relatively straightforward — expose the body to a small threat from the offending organism in the anticipation that the body will develop resistance and immunity by way of antibodies to then protect itself from a larger threat in the future. This concept is the basis for the majority of vaccinations in the world.

Smallpox was detected in Egyptian mummies from over 3000 years ago. It was identified as a huge world threat and vaccinations through inoculation were introduced in the late 18th century, continuing into the 20th century, when smallpox was officially eradicated. In the 19th century, rabies, typhoid, cholera and the plague were studied and then vaccinations developed. In the early 20th century, vaccinations for tuberculosis, diphtheria, influenza and tetanus were further studied and developed. In the latter 20th century, polio, measles, mumps, rubella, hepatitis and meningococcus vaccinations were added. Some examples of more recent 21st-century vaccines include those for herpes, new meningococcal strains, human papilloma virus and Japanese encephalitis.

The COVID-19 vaccination program set all-time records in relation to research, development and introduction of vaccines into the world medical marketplace due to the huge threat that COVID-19 delivered to the world on a global health and economic scale in 2020.

In Australia, a childhood immunisation schedule is offered to all families from birth. This covers vaccines for hepatitis B, diphtheria, tetanus, whooping cough, polio, pneumococcus and meningococcal strains. The introduction of these vaccines has been credited with significantly reducing infant and child mortality from these diseases. After 12 months, measles, mumps, rubella and chicken pox protection can be added to the program. Many education institutions require a child's immunisation to be up to date before they begin childcare, kindergarten or primary school.

During school years and adult life, various vaccination boosters are required to protect against common illness, such as influenza, pneumococcus, shingles (over 70 years) as well as boosters for conditions such as hepatitis, typhoid, cholera or tetanus, depending on occupation and travel requirements.

My message is again relatively simple: the overall history of vaccinations has shown that they have been protective against severe illness and death over the last 100 years and more. Unless significant contraindications emerge to vaccinations, they remain an important step in maintaining your health and ensuring that you address any potential causes of illness that may impact on the quality of your life and healthspan. As always, seek the advice of your healthcare professional, and discuss what vaccinations you require, your risk profile, and what eligibility you have.

HABITS

#69 Know your family history

I mention throughout this book the importance of knowing the various contributors and risk indicators when it comes to health or illness, and particularly those that may predict future health problems.

While many risk factors may need addressing, the three primary ones here are age, gender and family history.

While many of the other risk factors (such as smoking and poor nutrition) can be addressed by lifestyle changes, these three are the ones over which you have very little control. Unfortunately, the best medical care can't alter your birthdate and as you age, you can't avoid the fact you need to take better care of yourself. Time will march on. Similarly, gender is a fixed risk factor (with due respect to the transgender movement that is happening globally) and from an overall health risk perspective males seem to be more prone to a variety of health conditions and on a global basis have a shorter lifespan than women. Finally, family history relates to genetics (DNA) and is an absolutely critical factor in health prediction.

You need to be as aware of any medical conditions that regularly occur in your family background as possible. For example, in some families the incidence of cancers such as bowel, breast, prostate or skin is high. Similarly, heart disease, diabetes and lung problems may regularly occur, and this is related to the DNA and family background. The increased risk may come directly from parents (through the mother or father) or through aunts and uncles. Sometimes these conditions may even skip a generation and occur in the grandparents and then be passed onto grandchildren. While genetics is no longer thought to be as strong a determinant of future health risks as poor lifestyle choices, it still can account for 20 to 25 per cent of illness risk.

Clearly it is important to know if you are prone to any health risks based on your family background. If so, screening and testing can commence, usually at a younger age than those individuals who do not have any family background of these predictable conditions. As I have previously stated, so many of our common illnesses now have screening tests and, when detected early, the outcome and chances of long-term survival are dramatically improved.

By being aware of your family background, you can identify whether you need to have early check-ups for particular conditions—for example, a colonoscopy for bowel cancer or early breast screening for breast cancer. So don't pretend it won't happen to you if you don't talk about it. Find out your history, and discuss any known risks with your doctor. In this way, you can take control of your future and reduce the likelihood of more severe occurrences for these conditions. You will not only prolong your lifespan by doing so, but also improve your health throughout that journey to enjoy better quality of life as you head to 100 years and beyond!

HABITS

9
Mindset

Being open to change and evolution in your life is so important. Part of the skill of improving yourself, your overall outlook and your relationship with others is being prepared to consider, and potentially adopt, new things that may enhance your future, particularly from a health perspective.

In this chapter, I suggest some ways to enhance your personal development and learn from others. I hope you find inspiration among them.

Focus on yourself—and nurture others

Studies have shown a clear link between a positive mental state and improved health, including lower blood pressure, reduced risk of heart disease, healthier weight, better blood sugar levels and longer life.

An important part of improving your mental state is, of course, managing your stress and avoiding burnout. And I provide some strategies and tips in these areas in the following sections. A further sign of emotional wellness, however, is being able to hold onto positive emotions longer and appreciate the good times. Practising gratitude, developing a sense of meaning and purpose in life—and setting clear goals to help you focus on what's important to you—all contribute to emotional wellness. Further pieces in the puzzle are appreciating your relationship with others, practising compassion, and finding mentors, confidantes and experts.

All these aspects work together to improve your mental—and your physical—health. As ancient Greek philosopher Epicurus noted, 'The ultimate goal of the blessed life is physical health and mental serenity.'

#70 Manage your stress

I find the concept of stress a fascinating subject. I think everyone in the world understands the nebulous concept of stress and has probably experienced a period of time in their life when they have been 'under stress'. Even though the experience may be universal, the concept of being 'under stress' means vastly different things to different people and can manifest in a multitude of different ways—both physical and emotional. It intrigues me because it is an 'invisible' condition in some ways and has defied a clear definition despite many attempts by scientists, psychologists and other health practitioners.

The situations that commonly cause stress are perhaps easier to define. Perhaps you recognise some (or many) of the following:

- conflict

- financial pressure

- frustration

- health concerns

- lack of control

- life changes

- relationship issues

- uncertainty.

The preceding list is hardly exhaustive, and I could go on with many other examples. (Trust me, I have experienced them all!) While most people have probably experienced a number of these circumstances, the impact that they have on your system can vary widely. Working out how to deal with the stress that is imposed by these conditions is really the point I am aiming for in achieving a healthy life for you.

While the concept of stress is well known to most of us, it really only became popularised in the 1980s. Perhaps prior to that our parents, grandparents and great grandparents enjoyed a more relaxed style of life where stress was not a commonly used term as a feature of everyday survival in life—or perhaps they didn't talk about it as much. While it might seem that 'stress' is another negative condition of our modern society, the feelings it creates have been around for a long time.

The origins of stress

I was extremely surprised when researching this book to learn that, in the medical context, the term 'stress' was only first used

(continued)

in 1936. Medical doctor and endocrinologist Hans Selye first used the term, defining it in the medical context as 'the non-specific response of the body to any demand for change'. He based his findings on his experiments with rats, which he placed under extreme conditions such as freezing environments and high winds. He then observed the negative physiological changes that occurred in their body's organs, particularly their adrenal gland. The study of the body's physiological responses to stress, including cortisol production, was thus borne. Selye also worked with human patients and noted that, no matter what particular condition his hospitalised patients suffered from, they exhibited one common trait—they all became unwell with anxiety, high pulse rate and agitation. These are key points in the manifestations of stress in most human beings. (Prior to Selye's use of the word, the concept of stress was only applied in the engineering and construction context in relation to structural damage being caused to materials used in structures such as a bridge or high-rise building.)

Other historians dispute that Selye was the first to identify stress as a human physiological response. Psychology historians also credit Walter Cannon who, in his work relating to the development of the fight or flight response in 1915, also described stress. Importantly, psychologists distinguish between stress that is harmful (*distress*) and stress that can be positive (*eustress*). Positive stress embraces changes across biochemical, behavioural, physiological and psychological effects in the body.

In any event, while stress is something you are likely familiar with in your everyday language, it is in fact a relatively newly defined concept and one that is continuing to evolve with studies.

What does stress look like?

In one sense, stress is 'invisible'; however, it does have some commonly recognised manifestations. These can include the following:

- agitation

- catastrophising

- depersonalisation

- disconnection

- fear

- headaches

- hyperventilation

- increased heart rate

- irrational decision-making

- irritability

- muscle tension

- nausea

- nervousness

- overthinking

- panic attacks

- restlessness

- rumination

MINDSET

- second-guessing

- sleep disturbance

- social avoidance

- sweating

- tight chest

- trembling.

The ways that stress may manifest in an individual's behaviour are extraordinary, and the preceding list is far from exhaustive. You may also have your own suggestions to add.

Why is it that some individuals are very prone to stress reactions, yet others seem to sail through life with hardly a care in the world? While reactions and responses are likely greatly influenced by your upbringing, your own attitude and your sense of your ability to 'control' situations where stress may manifest are also vitally important.

As mentioned in the nearby breakout box, certain low levels of stress can actually create responses that are positive (eustress). In my time working with elite athletes, I have learnt that performance is best during an optimal level of arousal or nervousness — this leads to better focus and application to the task at hand.

Psychologists have also suggested that a small dose of stress can be a positive thing, whereby those who live and cope with small amounts of stress develop healthier habits such as avoiding excessive alcohol or other unhealthy choices such as smoking. When combined with a positive attitude towards life and high degree of emotional awareness, these traits contribute to healthy longevity.

Dealing with stress

Learning strategies to help with stress is extremely important. This might include taking a step back to look at the bigger picture in any tough situation, rather than getting buried in small issues and frustrations. Other useful strategies for 'in the moment' relief include breathing techniques, a short meditation and developing an ability to focus on something more important than the current stress situation. Even a brief 10-minute walk around the block can allow you to refocus.

This is not to say that you should ignore a circumstance where action is required to deal with an obstruction or negative event in your life. I am simply advocating having the tools available to know when a stressful situation is potentially presenting itself and how you will need to deal with it. Life stress does lead to many individuals gaining the resources required, often through trial and error and the experience of the negative outcomes from their past.

TIP

To help deal with stressful situations over the long term, adopt ongoing relaxation strategies. These might include regular yoga and meditation, taking regular time out for yourself to do something you love (including exercise), seeking social support or connecting with others. Recognising the early signs of an impending stress situation and taking action to avoid the escalation of that situation is a significant help.

One of the major clinical areas for psychologists is helping individuals deal with the anxiety and panic that is associated with stress in their lives. Techniques such as cognitive behaviour therapy are often utilised.

At times, certain medications may also be prescribed to try to stabilise the chemical imbalance that can be associated with the stress hormones going haywire. In most circumstances, this is a short-term intervention to help the individual regain relaxing sleep patterns and function in their day-to-day activities without the distraction of anxiety, irritability, tremor or high heart rates, all of which are physiological manifestations of the body being out of balance.

Exercise (my favourite!) is also an important therapeutic tool for stress management. This is because exercise can:

- enhance your mood (through neurochemical release)

- boost self esteem

- allow for social interaction

- promote teamwork and goal setting

- improve sleep

- reduce tension

- build relationships

- be enjoyable (through the release of 'happy hormones' — refer to chapter 8).

The concept of stress is not news to anyone; however, how it manifests or is described can be much more challenging. The secret is being able to deal with a stressful situation through your own behaviour techniques, and working to ensure stress doesn't have an impact on our health going forward. Otherwise, it will be an inhibitor to you achieving your long healthy life.

#71 Recognise and avoid burnout

....

You've likely heard the term 'burnout' used at some stage in your life. While it can take many forms, burnout generally involves an individual losing motivation and becoming both physically and emotionally detached from the particular activity they are engaged in. In many situations, this applies to a career or occupation where an individual simply loses motivation and interest in their work, which can obviously then affect performance in a substantial way. Poor or irrational decision-making can result.

Defining burnout can be controversial. The formal definition of burnout generally relates to a syndrome associated with chronic workplace stress that has become overwhelming. It is often characterised by increasing mental distancing from your occupation together with feelings of inadequacy and exhaustion as well as negativity or cynicism towards your job. Burnout is a state of emotional, physical and mental exhaustion occurring when you feel overwhelmed or unable to meet the constant demands and stress associated with your situation, usually your work occupation. While it can occur at different levels of severity, the most significant forms of burnout result in an individual having to change their occupation in order to protect their future health. However, it manifests in many different ways in each individual experiencing burnout.

Certainly, burnout is much more frequently discussed in today's society than it was in the past. I know of many individuals who were experiencing lack of motivation and disenchantment with their occupation but probably did not realise that they were going through a burnout phase at that time. While some people may recover from burnout and persist in the same direction, industry or career they were previously in, more often people have to reprogram themselves and change to a different direction in life. Admitting to burnout used to have a stigma attached to it, but in these days of greater consciousness and awareness of mental health disorders, burnout has become more accepted and has less stigma attached. Nonetheless, I am sure people continue to struggle significantly with their situation, undergoing true burnout but are not able to recognise the situation or not prepared to do something about it. Perhaps some still consider it a sign of weakness to submit to the burnout stress and so continue to push on in the workplace or other environments to the detriment of their own personal health as well as their performance.

In this context, I am not talking about simply having a few bad days in your life where things do not go well. In most circumstances, this is a temporary situation and is simply part of the highs and lows of life that we all must experience. You can recover from this. However, true burnout is more chronic in nature and can build up over a much more substantial period, not just a few days. The trick is being able to recognise the signs in yourself and then seeking intervention to sort this out. This might be simply a matter of talking to your superiors in your workplace to make some changes to your work environment to allow you to refresh. In other circumstances, you might require more professional outside psychological assistance to deal with any deep-seated issues.

The world is now full of many examples of individuals who have experienced extreme burnout in their past careers but have moved on to an even more successful life after reprogramming themselves through a change for the better. This may include looking after their health in a much more active way than they had done in the past. Bookshop shelves are loaded with self-help books focused on this area, many written by those who have experienced burnout in their own circumstances.

> **TIP**
>
> If you feel you are experiencing burnout, have a look through the shelves at your local bookshop and find an expert author whose approach appeals to you. You can also seek professional help from the many psychologists who now specialise in this field.

You need to look after yourself from both an emotional and physical health point of view. All too often people who have experienced burnout have put others ahead of themselves — including family and workmates — and that has resulted in a negative impact on their own personal situation. (See later in this chapter for more on being selfish and why it's not always a bad thing.)

If you know someone who is going through burnout symptoms or recognise it in yourself, make sure you seek help and make the changes before it becomes a chronic issue for you in life.

#72 Build your willpower (and avoid the 'won't power')

I think 'willpower' is a term that most of us have used at some stage in our lives. While it probably means different things in different circumstances, the general assumption is that it refers to your ability to make a tough decision and act accordingly, particularly in circumstances where it may have some slightly unpleasant ramifications. For example, when someone is talking about their desire to lose weight, they will often say something like, 'I really would like to lose weight, but I lack the willpower to do so.' Unfortunately, willpower is very much an internal characteristic and, apart from the encouragement that someone might obtain from outside individuals such as friends and colleagues, the ultimate choice as to how to make that decision comes down to the individual.

I remember when I was a youngster in primary school growing up in Geelong. The parish priest at our local church, St Margaret's in East Geelong, was Father Neville McKay. He was an avid football follower and a great fan of the Carlton Football Club ('the Blues'). I distinctly remember many of his Sunday morning sermons referred to how Carlton had performed the previous day in its football match. Needless to say, his sermons were both entertaining as well as educational. To me, he stood out as a shining light at a time when many priests presented quite a serious side and rarely engaged in conversation that was relatable to an eight year old.

Neville (as he asked me to call him) was also a habitual smoker. His usual consumption was around 20 to 25 cigarettes per day, and he rarely did any exercise. Even at that young age, I sometimes had conversations with him around exercise and health and he told me how he would dearly love to give up smoking but wasn't able to do so. I mentioned to him at the time that it was probably a matter of 'willpower'. Remember—willpower was something young catholic boys were being asked to exhibit as part of our traditional upbringing. I thought I could get back at him by challenging him with the same request!

His response to me was, 'Pete, I have lots of willpower. Unfortunately, what I don't have is any "won't power"!' This quote has remained with me throughout my entire life, and I have often quoted Father Neville when speaking to patients who are trying to make a decision regarding lifestyle changes and the topic of their willpower (or lack thereof) arises. In the context that Neville used the phrase, it was quite apt. We often want to make choices that involve us excluding a certain item from our lives, or stopping an unhealthy behaviour — be it smoking, poor nutrition, lack of exercise, anger management or impatience. The decision to avoid the 'won't power' attitude and replace it with the positive step to make the change is absolutely critical in assisting with internal decision-making to improve your life. So next time you are discussing your inability to make a change and blaming it on lack of willpower, remember Neville (as I frequently do) and make the decision to improve yourself.

Here are some examples of key challenges:

- 'I won't continue to smoke on a daily basis.'

- 'I won't continue to delay my exercise program.'

- 'I won't keep consuming high-fat sugary treats on a frequent basis.'

Remember, it's up to you — you are the one in control of your decision-making.

#73 Don't be too hard on yourself

Many of us go through periods in our lives where we feel down and unhappy with our situation. It may be that we have made mistakes through work or other circumstances in life, or perhaps have not achieved a goal that we have set out in our overall health program.

While self-reflection and learning from mistakes is valuable, it's also important not to be too hard on yourself. Being too negative can sometimes result in you giving up on your goals completely. Instead, recognise the small gains you have made and continue to set targets.

Be prepared to reward yourself for the small gains because these will accumulate over time.

It is also important to realise that the pathway to achieving improvement is not always perfect, straight or progressive. You will experience setbacks, troughs and dips on this path that can challenge your commitment. You need to refocus and readjust at these times and just set yourself a small achievable goal. It is okay to praise yourself when you then reach this goal because doing so will reinforce that you are capable of making the progress you desire. Being continuously hard on yourself creates negative feedback and does have an impact on your brain's neurochemical balance.

Be positive and you will see the results.

#74 Think like a child

Now, I am not suggesting here that you regress to your childhood behaviour of tantrums and always wanting to get your own way. (Although that is a tactic some of my adult friends adopt when they are trying to prove a point!) What I am referring to here is the amazing ability young children have to simplify matters in life and adopt a clarity that is often lacking as we progress through our development years.

I do not think you need to be a parent to understand how amazing young children can be in the way they see the world; however, from my own perspective, becoming a parent certainly opened my eyes more fully. If you work in childcare, kindergartens and early learning centres, you will have made the same observations that I am referring to here.

Children have a way of seeing joy and fun in everything they do. Of course, they also experience frustrations as they learn the basics of life, but those who have been parents get to witness on a regular basis the joy and fun that children see in so much of what they do.

As we grow older in life, we tend to narrow our focus and change the way we see things — and perhaps overanalyse situations. What has amazed me in dealing with children from as young as two or three years is the way they see the world in such a simplistic way and don't overcomplicate matters. My young son was observing a beautiful blue summer sky with a few wispy white clouds. He asked me if clouds could fly because they didn't fall out of the sky like other objects he threw up in the air. Brilliant!

Obviously, our adult thoughts become muddled by life experiences, expectations of what we think should be the right thing to do, and perhaps our biased educational and learning experiences. Young children, on the other hand, simply use their intuition and spontaneous interpretation of situations in life. They will speak up without all the congested background brain experience and biases that adults clog their thought processes with. A child will often only see the positive aspects of a situation in life. Their giggles and cheerful laughter are a highlight of some of my early parenting. The sheer joy of such simple things as blowing bubbles, playing with a pet kitten or puppy and frolicking in the shallow waters on the beach are really what enjoying life should be all about. If only we, as adults, could shed that external veneer and revel in the simple pleasures of rolling in the grass, jumping on a jumping castle and appreciating some of the simplest jokes of all time.

So, without reverting to your negative childhood behaviours, simply reflect on the joy and pleasures that young children bring to the world. And maybe try to emulate some of those simple enjoyments

MINDSET

now and as you age, rather than leaving them behind in your early
development years.

#75 Practise gratefulness

You've no doubt been exposed to the phrase 'be grateful for what
you have' (or something similar). Generally, this advice is given to
us by an elder or a mentor at a time when we may be lamenting our
position in life and when things are not going well for us. It may take
us all some time to develop an appreciation for this advice, but it
usually rings true!

Many studies now confirm that practising gratefulness is actually a
way to a better life. However, it is not as easy as it sounds. Getting
caught up in what we are doing in life and not appreciating what
we already have is all too easy. It is a challenge for many to accept
that we all need to learn to be grateful for the things that we already
have achieved rather than coveting things that we do not have or are
inaccessible to us. I am not just speaking of material things, such as
clothes, cars and beach houses, but the most important things we
have in lives, such as our friends, family and health. Nevertheless,
I believe it is in our human make-up to naturally observe others
around us and, from time to time, compare them with ourselves.

Many of you will be familiar with the phrase 'the grass is always
greener on the other side'. While this saying can be traced back as
far as the poetry of Ovid (43 BCE–17 CE), its modern interpretation
can be applied to many circumstances. (Ovid is actually credited with
stating, *'fertilior seges est alenis semper in agris'* — the harvest is always
more fruitful in another man's fields.) In any event, the meaning is
most likely obvious to all of you — most of us are prone to wanting

something that we do not have, all the while not appreciating that where we are and what we have is actually pretty good.

People who practise gratefulness have been shown to be more content and are more likely to be productive in their life. The benefits flow on to a healthier existence from both a physical and emotional point of view. Studies have shown that feeling more grateful can improve sleep, mood and immunity, and also reduce depression, anxiety, difficulties with chronic pain and risk of disease.

So, it is important to look around and see what you have in your life — and not necessarily your material possessions — and appreciate them for the good that they bring to your life. By being aware of this, you are less likely to stress over unachievable or fanciful options that may not even be appropriate to your circumstances. In fact, things that appear attractive from a distance may actually be far less appealing when you know the inside story. That green grass can turn out to be fake and artificial!

> ## *TIP*
> Once you learn to practise gratefulness (gratitude), you will be more content internally and have added another strategy on your path to a long and happy life.

#76 Be selfish — it's not always a bad choice!

From our earliest days, most of us were taught that the word 'selfish' was a negative term and a type of behaviour we should avoid. However, I want to emphasise that the importance of looking after one's 'self' should never be underestimated, and is a critical part of maintaining your health profile.

How often do we hear an individual say, 'I'm too busy to exercise, meditate, take a break (etcetera, etcetera)'? Those individuals who are too absorbed by work, careers, meetings and other life tasks often falsely believe they are being committed and loyal to their business, job, family finances or whatever it is that makes them so 'busy'. They even justify their stance by imagining they are preparing and setting themselves up for the 'future' — all the while not recognising they are exhausting themselves in the present.

It is easy to convince yourself that you have so many others depending on you that you cannot slow down.

My question to you in this situation is a simple one: 'What would happen if you were not here?' What if you had a serious heart attack? Or died? What would your family do? What would your business or family finances be like? Looking after yourself, and keeping yourself healthy and productive, means you are looking after those people who depend on you also.

By putting yourself first for a change (even briefly) — that is, being 'selfish' about your health — you are actually doing more for your family, business, employees and others than by burning out and becoming more unhealthy every year. Each of us only has 168 hours in our week. If you achieve the target of 150 minutes per week of moderately vigorous exercise time (refer to chapter 6), you are actually only committing around 1.5 per cent of your week to personal health through physical activity. What an investment! That's a very small allocation for a huge upside in health and longevity returns.

Taking time for our own self is important. In my mind, this is the true meaning of the word selfish in the health preservation sense — allocating some 'self' time to make sure you are being the best you can be. This often means taking some time to exercise, relax, meditate or simply gain that personal space that allows you to unwind and remove yourself from the pressures of everyday living. In this way, you are committing personal time to truly looking after yourself and really redefining the importance of what it means to be selfish. Giving yourself this personal investment adds another strategy in your path to a healthy and successful long life.

#77 Never stop learning

One of the great things about the modern world is that new things are always being discovered and being put in front of us to challenge our beliefs and past habits. I believe it is important to keep an open mind to all these things and to be prepared to make changes, especially in a positive way, to promote healthy living and a more comfortable healthy life. If you have a closed mind and are not willing to make changes as you age, you're more likely to be stuck with poor lifestyle habits and will thus fail to embrace new concepts that may assist you in your health journey.

While many new ideas and strategies may not be totally appropriate for every individual, those that have validated research supporting them should be considered. The important thing is being receptive to these ideas. It might be as simple as understanding the value of a food type that you have traditionally not used in your cooking or had on your weekly shopping list. Friends may suggest a new healthy vegetable they have found. (Kale made an appearance in my house in 2020 — I'm still adapting!) Often these changes can be easily incorporated into everyday living. By keeping an open mind to new ideas and new concepts, you continually rejuvenate and regenerate yourself so you can be the best version of yourself.

MINDSET

So next time you hear of a new idea or concept that is perhaps foreign to your past experiences, do not automatically dismiss it outright. Give some consideration as to whether it may have some merit. While some new ideas may not suit you individually, others can be adapted.

Remember — we are all victims of our past experiences and biases. I know I have personally sometimes closed myself to new ideas in the past because they did not fit with my normal habitual behaviour, or my fixed concepts of the way things should be done in my world. On many occasions, after some consideration (and wisdom of experience), I have come to understand that these new concepts had merit and, subsequently, they have become part of my everyday behaviours. As an example, controlled slow breathing was not something I had thought about, or practised, until recent years. It is now part of my repertoire, and something I can reach for as needed. Thus, I have convinced myself that even I can keep learning at my stage of my career and life journey. I'm sure the same is true for you.

#78 Set your goals

One of the most important ways to organise your life and create a structure that allows you to introduce healthy lifestyle changes is to create a list of goals for yourself. These can be simple tasks that you want to get done on a daily or weekly basis, or even over a more extended period of time (for example, annual targets). It is important to divide your challenges or goals into small achievable stages (for example, weight loss of two kilograms per month) so that you can see the rewards over a period of time. Small simple achievements lead to larger cumulative goal achievements.

I have worked in elite sport for many decades. I can guarantee you that highly successful athletes are usually very structured in the way they lay out their goals for what they want to achieve. They divide these target goals into smaller steps and then they follow their plan to progress to the end goal.

In my time dealing with successful elite athletes, these are some of the traits that I believe have led to them achieving their goals:

- They possess a natural hunger and drive.

- They possess strong discipline — for example, with training, sleep and nutrition.

- They make sacrifices — particularly when it comes to aspects such as their social life.

- They set high expectations — elite athletes are usually their best critics (and most harsh on themselves).

- They aim high — someone has to be the best, so why not make it yourself?

- They possess internal belief — they want to achieve the changes and believe they can, although they know they will be frequently challenged.

- They set firm goals.

- They divide the process into small achievable stages — encouragement comes from small gains.

- They understand it is not an easy path and, therefore, prepare for and expect setbacks.

MINDSET

- They demonstrate resilience — every elite athlete has a story of failure or setback that they have overcome in order to return to their plan and achieve their ultimate goals.

You don't need to be a sportsperson (or even a sports lover) to appreciate these. And while you don't need to emulate every one of these traits in a strict sense, this list gives you an indication of some of the principles you can apply. You can then plan your own changes that you are willing to make and set your own goals with respect to your lifestyle in order to progress towards the achievable healthy 100 years and beyond.

> ### TIP
> Achieving your goals starts with wanting to improve yourself and creating the best environment for you to be as productive in life as you can. Small changes introduced consistently soon become lifestyle habits, which then facilitate longer term benefits. Goal setting then becomes yet another strategy for you to be your best in your life journey.

The little achievements also give you a burst of your 'happy hormones' such as dopamine. Get to it — make those plans!

#79 Pay attention to the detail

One of the themes of this book is me reminding you to be prepared and organised during your busy week. This can include planning your exercise sessions, implementing a good sleep schedule, and building in time for food shopping as well as personal care and development. During my time in international sport at a competitive level, I came across many successful athletes who I would categorise as eccentric or obsessive. This was one of the characteristic traits of most of the gold medallists and world record holders I met, and being highly organised probably helped give them an edge.

I certainly don't think that having an obsessive-compulsive personality disorder (OCD) is a healthy way to live in most circumstances, but being an organised person does help. This is what I refer to as ATD (attention to detail). Having an organised ATD life is not the same as being obsessive or compulsive. It simply means you are giving yourself the best opportunity to organise your time efficiently.

Making sure you line up the little things in your life, whether it be through making a list or having a well-organised diary, means that you can plan and keep track of the important things you need to cover in the time ahead. Focusing on the detail may be as simple as maintaining a regular healthy shopping list, planning good sleep hygiene in your bedroom, or organising the correct components of your exercise program to cover the cardio, strength and flexibility aspects that are important.

I know, at times, close friends and colleagues have spoken to me about my commitment to my work, exercise or general lifestyle. They say something to me along the lines of, 'I am impressed by how obsessive you are about that.' My response to them is that it is not about obsession, it is simply about my ATD. I am certainly not claiming that I get it correct all the time. However, at least having a good intention most of the time means that I can juggle all the important things and make the most of the time available to optimise efficiency from a work productivity, as well as personal health management perspective.

Where do you fit in the spectrum? Getting some of the small details right will allow you to move forward in your planning of a well-organised, long and healthy living plan.

MINDSET

#80 Avoid
.... procrastination

I was going to write this section much sooner but, unfortunately, I put off doing so. Seriously, I am only kidding, but if I look at my past, I would have to admit to being one of the greatest procrastinators I know. Probably in gold medal class if I'm really honest with myself!

Procrastination is the art of putting off a decision or an action until another time. One of the great procrastination sayings of all time is 'I'll get around to it'. (I was once sent a photo of a 'round tuit'—it was a round non-descript object. This, of course, was a humorous attempt by someone to highlight how frequently the phrase was used in society. Clearly, a round tuit doesn't exist, but you get my point!)

Usually, it is the hard decisions or difficult tasks in life over which we all procrastinate. Making a decision to go ahead with something that is appealing or easy to achieve, even on a daily basis, is much easier than tackling the hard tasks. However, I have found this only creates more stress in relation to making the hard decision and delays the inevitable.

One strategy I have found useful, particularly as I have improved my procrastination behaviour in recent years, is to make a list of tasks that are required for that day, week or month and then prioritise based on how important they are. Then I will often rate them according to which are the easiest to achieve and which are the most difficult for me personally. Often, the easy task is less important, but it is the one that our human nature behaviour leads us to tackle first.

As I have grown better at not putting off the difficult tasks, I have found it useful to tackle the most difficult tasks at the beginning of my 'to-do list' instead of the simple, non-important things that really can wait until another time. In this way, I have found that the satisfaction from completing a difficult task (particularly one I have procrastinated over for way too long) is much more rewarding than the satisfaction from completing the simple, less-important tasks. I'm far from perfect at achieving this goal every time, but I have made the changes in my behaviour and recognise the emotional lift I get from completing the harder challenge.

Sometimes simply remembering the feeling that comes from completing a difficult task is enough to make you realise you should undertake other difficult tasks sooner. Not only will you get the task completed, but you will also avoid the discomfort of putting it off, stressing about when it is going to get done and then putting yourself under unnecessary pressure to complete it with an impending deadline.

Frequently, I would put a task off until the night before it was due. So, while I always had faith in myself to complete the task (even if it meant staying up all night to do so), inevitably this approach only delayed the satisfaction of completing the task and usually did not leave enough time to revise the final outcome, if required. I realise that not everyone is a world champion procrastinator as I used to be, but I think we can all relate to avoiding unpleasant tasks in the hope that they can be done at some other time.

My advice for improving your life is to try to avoid delaying tackling the difficult situations (particularly those which inevitably have to be done anyway) and try to allocate time to get them done. This is another important tip in improving your life and avoiding unnecessary stress. (There—I've got this section done!! Insert self-congratulations here!)

MINDSET

#81 Learn the value of solitude

....

In the next chapter, I outline the importance of social connectivity and integration in your healthy lifestyle. However, on some occasions we all need some solo personal space. The ability to seek out some peaceful time on your own for meditation, reflection and creative thinking cannot be underestimated.

We all lead busy lives, and on occasion we all need to get away from the true hustle and bustle — whether that be work, family or other commitments — and simply have some 'alone time'. (This is similar to the idea of being selfish — see earlier in this chapter.)

Seeking out solitude need not be for a lengthy period of time. You may simply want some alone time for a single evening, a day or a weekend away. This break allows you to gather your thoughts and have some time to reflect on where you are in your life journey. This can allow you to reset your goals and priorities for the time ahead.

Sometimes it is important to roster yourself a day off — a mental health day — so you can explore that personal time and catch up with anything you may not otherwise get to during the hectic other parts of your week.

Finding this time for yourself can assist with your mental health stability and allow you to refresh before returning to your normal commitments. Planning some solitary time should be a component of your overall direction when creating your healthy lifestyle moving forward. This is a health behaviour that took some time for me to appreciate — I was always 'too busy' to slow down. Since I adopted it on a regular basis, I have seen a massive difference in my emotional balance and work productivity.

#82 Practise compassion

Compassion literally means 'to suffer together'. In reality, it means extending sympathy, empathy or concern for others who are experiencing misfortune or some other negative experience in their life. The ability to be compassionate towards others is a great characteristic and is another step in developing your personality and creating a more balanced life. Understanding the suffering of others and being able to assist in their time of need can also be an advantage when you are personally experiencing a difficult emotional event.

It really is not that hard to extend assistance to an individual who is in need. This might be as simple as helping someone in the street who requires assistance crossing the road or carrying some heavy shopping bags to their car. Perhaps it could be reaching out to someone you know when you hear that they have experienced some difficult event in their life. The individuals to whom you show compassion do not necessarily have to be close friends or family — they could simply be an acquaintance or someone in the same workplace, even if you do not know them well.

When you provide some compassionate support for other people, you may experience a sense of calmness or wellbeing yourself that contributes to your own health situation. Compassion does not necessarily have to be a specific action but can be more related to showing some emotional support by way of conversation or just keeping company for someone in their time of need. Just the basic act of enquiring how someone is going at a difficult time can lift their spirit and have more impact than you might realise. A simple effort can make a big difference to someone's day — and it may provide you with some important new perspective on your own stage in life.

MINDSET

If you are able to introduce compassion into your day-to-day behaviours you have taken another step along the pathway to a healthy, more fulfilling and productive life.

#83 Seek out mentors

By definition, a mentor is an experienced or trusted advisor who can assist you with a whole range of stages of your life. Sometimes, mentors come into our lives without us seeking them out, and sometimes they are right under our noses by way of contacts we have in our everyday activities.

A mentor might be as obvious as a teacher at school, a neighbour or relative who took a special interest in your upbringing, or someone in your workplace who took you under their wing and continues to advise you going forward. Being receptive to this advice and guidance is a critical part of your learning process and understanding how you can be your best self.

In the traditional medical world, mentors tend to be more experienced colleagues with whom one may be working. This might be either in the hospital setting, where junior doctors have a senior unit leader, or perhaps in a more specialised medical training program, with a guiding consultant specialist.

No doubt you can look back at periods of your life and recognise that certain individuals (usually older than yourself) had an influence on you, even if at the time you may not have considered them to have the formal title of mentor.

A mentor does not necessarily have to be someone with whom you spend a lot of time but is usually someone you respect and follow in their career or lifestyle, learning from their behaviours and example. Sometimes, you may simply aspire to be like that person, using their behaviour and achievements as a way of setting your own goals. In other circumstances, the mentor may be someone that you have a lot of direct contact with and can seek out with direct questioning, conversation and 'coaching sessions' to assist you with difficult decisions or stages of your life and career.

Regardless of the field of work you are in, mentors will be available who you can seek out and gain help with whatever you are requiring. Modern technology now means you can have such instant communication via email or video conferencing, and even more ease of travel these days means you can spend time with business leaders in their field and seek their guidance. I wish I had had these technologies available to me when I was setting out in my career.

Perhaps you're reluctant to approach high-profile individuals in the belief that they will not have time for you and be too busy to give you assistance. However, I encourage you to simply make the approach—you might be surprised how receptive they are. I have been fortunate in my career to meet and deal with some very high-profile individuals in Australia and elsewhere—not just in medicine or sport but also significant international business leaders—and I have found every one of them to be approachable and willing to talk to young individuals.

MINDSET

> ### *TIP*
> Be brave, ask the hard questions and seek out someone you admire—you might be surprised how receptive and generous with their time they are. Your life path will be enhanced in ways you might not have imagined.

My own personal mentors

When I look back at my own early days in my sports medicine career, unfortunately very few individuals—and therefore potential mentors—were working in the field I hoped to pursue. However, I definitely had people who guided me along the way.

I remember our family general practitioner in Geelong, Dr Kevin Threlfall, who spent most of his time working as a dedicated family care doctor but also had a side interest working with sporting teams, including the Geelong Football Club in the Victorian Football League (VFL). Kevin became my 'go-to' doctor when I had a sports injury as a young athlete at age 11 or 12. (Fortunately, I did not have too many injuries that Kevin needed to sort out!) Kevin also became president of the Geelong Football Club and reactivated the VFL Doctors Association, of which I was a young junior member. I thought he had a great blended medical and sport mix in his lifestyle.

Similarly at age 17, I was fortunate to meet Dr Howard Toyne when I was attending an athletics competition meeting at Olympic Park stadium. Howard was an experienced surgeon in Melbourne but he had a great interest in sport, particularly cycling and athletics. When I learned that he was the first doctor ever chosen to accompany an Australian Olympic Team to an Olympic Games (Tokyo 1964), I thought to myself, *What a cool job.* Almost at that point, I decided I wanted to be like Howard and follow in his career direction. He was kind enough to give me time on many occasions and indeed became my sports care doctor in my own athletics career when I moved to Melbourne at age 17 to attend university. When he retired, he gave me some of his office medical equipment, including his favourite patient examination couch—a possession I still use and treasure to this day.

Howard was well connected with overseas doctors as a result of his international experience. In particular, he had connections in the Eastern Bloc including Russia and East Germany, something that was extraordinarily unusual for an Australian doctor at that time, given the secrecy associated with elite sport in those nations. He set up introductions for me with the Olympic team doctor for the East German athletics team, based in Leipzig. Even at that time, I realised what a privilege that was for me.

He and I spoke regularly about the lack of opportunity to be trained as a sports medicine doctor in Australia. I clearly remember Howard telling me around 1975 that he believed a post graduate sports medicine course would be soon available in Australia for young doctors. He even predicted that this course might be available to me once I graduated from medical school in 1978. Unfortunately, Howard's predictions did not come to fruition, although I know he made several attempts with government to try to have a training institute set up—including at the St George's Hospital in Cotham Road, Kew. When I look back now with pride at the advances sports medicine has made in Australia, including having our own specialist college (the Australasian College of Sport and Exercise Physicians) which has a four-year post-graduate training program for doctors, I still think of Howard and how he would also be so proud that sports medicine has achieved what it has in Australia.

(The Australasian College of Sport and Exercise Physicians was established in 1985 but did not grant fellowship qualifications until 1991 and did not achieve federal government recognition as a specialty until 2011. I was a founding member in 1985 and received my foundation fellowship with the first group who passed their exams in 1991.)

MINDSET

(continued)

Back in the 1970s and early 1980s, I realised I would need to travel overseas if I wanted to pursue my goal of training to be a full-time sports medicine specialist. I was extremely fortunate to receive the inaugural Sir Robert Menzies travelling fellowship in 1982. This award allowed me to spend time overseas with a number of other extremely important mentors in my sports medicine pathway. (By way of perspective, the Menzies trust fellowship granted me £5000 for the entire year to travel—equivalent to AU$7500 at that time. I hardly lived the high life during that post-grad experience!)

While overseas, I sought out two exceptional individuals in Dr Doug Clement and Dr Jack Taunton at the University of British Columbia in Vancouver, both former high-achieving athletes and, at that stage, doctors with the Canadian Olympic Team. In my travels, I also met Dr Lyle Micheli, a Boston orthopaedic surgeon who specialised in children's sports injuries and who was based at Harvard University Children's Hospital. Lyle also inspired me to be interested in children's sports injuries and taught me a great deal about the resilience and recovery of young athletes. Dr John King in London and Dr Bill Garrick in San Francisco also kindly hosted me during that incredible year of research and learning.

On a more local level in Australia, Dr Ken Fitch was one of the most senior Australian Olympic Team doctors and my doctor for my first Olympic Team selection at the 1976 Montreal Olympic Games. Ken was based in Perth, Western Australia, and I was able to spend part of my fifth-year medical school elective study break in Perth under Ken's guidance. While a formal sports medicine course wasn't available at that time in Australia, I was still able to spend time at Shenton Park Rehabilitation Hospital and Sir Charles Gairdner Hospital in their trauma and orthopaedics departments. I also attended

Ken's practice where he was working particularly with Australian Rules football teams from East Perth and Claremont. Ken subsequently went on to serve many years as the doctor for the West Coast Eagles in the Australian Football League (AFL). Ken was also highly influential in the anti-doping scene both in Australia and at the IOC level, and was an advisor on the IOC doping commission as well as to the Australian anti-doping agencies. Ken nurtured and inspired me to maintain my interest in the world of doping in sport and is one of the individuals who encouraged me to continue my firm advocacy for anti-doping controls in elite sport.

These are the mentors I've been lucky enough to have over my years of training and development. Fortunately, these days young sports medicine doctors have a far greater pool of experienced specialists both in Australia and internationally from which they can seek guidance.

#84 Scrutinise expert opinion

One of the difficulties in navigating all the information about health behaviours is dealing with the conflicting evidence that regularly appears, endorsed by so-called industry experts. It can be quite confusing for the general consumer when a particular research paper or study is released that highlights an important health behaviour, only for that behaviour to be refuted the next day by a different industry expert who provides the opposite opinion.

Over the years, much information has been distributed and published on so many topics — such as the importance of low-fat (or high-fat) diets, the correct consumption of caffeine, and the amount of exercise one needs for health benefits. And this is without even entering the book shops that are totally bulging with publications giving advice on health and weight loss.

Inevitably, the consumer (that's you and me!) can be overwhelmed by the amount of information available, let alone by the need to interpret what is correct and what is false. Unfortunately, this will always be the case in the field of scientific studies, as you really have to drill down into the validity of many of these studies before determining whether the advice being delivered is truly accurate. For example, many studies are performed on subjects from one particular gender or age group and the findings may not apply to others. In other circumstances, certain racial variations in response to health behaviours may exist which do not apply across the world globally. The number of subjects in the study, duration of the study and how the conclusions are ultimately reached may all be criticised by independent research analysts. Sometimes researchers take considerable license in drawing their conclusions from their study and apply a more generalised advice statement that is really not appropriate based on the findings of the study when it is carefully dissected.

Genuine and valid scientific studies usually require a control group as well as a double-blind random allocation of interventions to make them legitimate in the medical and health world. Sadly, this is often not the case when the study has been funded by conflicted manufacturers that are endeavouring to have their product publicised by funding the study. This is known in my industry as 'research bias' and is unfortunately all too common. Findings can be further compromised when the study is performed in their own institution by their own employees. Those results need to be interpreted with a great deal of scrutiny and reliably repeated before being accepted in mainstream health advice.

Determining the accuracy of many of these studies can become a minefield, particularly in the absence of a regulatory body controlling the publicity that can be derived from certain products. Fortunately, in Australia the Therapeutic Goods Administration (TGA) has a firm control on medically based products. However, this is not the case with many of the nutrition products available in the marketplace because they do not qualify as 'medicines' or 'drugs' and so are not subject to TGA guidelines.

So, next time you hear of the latest wonder product or treatment, look carefully at the origin of the information being distributed as well as the medium in which it is being publicised—for example, a current affairs TV show. The latest 'scientific breakthrough' may not be all it seems. Testimonials and endorsements by celebrities or 'influencers' do not constitute legitimate evidence for the accuracy of the claims. Check on the TGA website (www.tga.gov.au) for any information currently available, and look for further studies backing up the findings of the study being publicised.

Finding your religion

This book is certainly not meant to be spiritual or religious in any evangelistic way. However, religion has been a great support to many people. For these people, their faith can assist them in times of need—whether that faith is Islam, Hinduism, Christianity or any of the many other faiths. Many different circumstances in life can mean people are undergoing a very difficult time, and religion can be the fallback to provide solace and comfort.

Perhaps during the death of a loved one, or some other major hurdle in life, you might find yourself returning to your faith to give you strength. Chatting with your faith's elder, priest,

(continued)

MINDSET

273

imam, rabbi, chaplain or other spiritual adviser can provide a perspective from another supportive angle.

Hopefully, you also have many other support systems around you, whether these are family or close friends, but you may also find your faith provides a solid grounding at times of reflection and troubles.

I grew up in an era when the Catholic education I received was very strict and formalised. Yet, I still recall religion providing a great source of solace for some of my older relatives at times when they lost partners or close friends. I also remember attending funerals as a youngster and, while the significance of the event was not lost on me, I perhaps didn't appreciate how much religion served as a support to the families involved.

Overcoming grief is something we all face, usually on many occasions in our life journey. So, while I'm not by any means pushing a religious direction, I am simply pointing out the great source of emotional relief and insight at difficult times having—or returning to—a faith can be. Having this support can help stabilise and reset your emotional balance and assist with moving forward in life with a healthy perspective. Do what feels right for you.

#85 Get a good financial planner

Now you might wonder why I am adding this as one of my health and fitness tips. Certainly, it is not strictly a health tip, but you will see why it is important in your overall life plan.

Firstly, we all need to recognise that we may need access to financial resources for unexpected injuries or illness-related costs later in life.

I would add that these costs may be greater for you if you do not follow the rest of the advice in this book! One thing I can say for certain is that the cost of health care in Australia has been increasing year by year and, if you need to access private care and don't have private health insurance to cover your medical needs, it can be a very expensive exercise. Couple this with the fact that the waiting times for many elective procedures in the Australian public healthcare system can be extraordinarily long, you will hopefully appreciate that having some financial resources to assist with unexpected health costs makes a lot of sense.

More importantly, however, the reason I am suggesting you need a good financial planner and accountant in your life is to make sure you have a solid nest egg of money available to enjoy your potential long life and healthspan. You should be planning ahead for this longer life and what finances you will need to truly enjoy it — perhaps to travel, take holidays, eat out, go on cruises or whatever other pleasures in life you hope to enjoy.

If you follow my advice to remain fit and active at 100 years of age and beyond, you will need these resources to keep up your enjoyable activities — and keep achieving your daily DOSE of happy hormones (refer to chapter 8).

Certainly, I did not appreciate the importance of good financial planning when I was starting out in my career. Of course, I had heard about superannuation and retirement investments but, as the years have passed, I have really come to appreciate the importance of these in obtaining financial security for the future. The traditional retirement age of 65 years (or in some industries 60 years) seems quite ludicrous in the modern era, given the regular skills shortages in the workplace and the amount of experience and intellectual property (IP) knowledge that people over 60 years of age possess. It may have been appropriate for our parents and grandparents to retire before

MINDSET

the age of 65, but certainly their expected lifespan (and healthspan) was not as it is in modern times.

I know of many individuals who thought they had enough money put aside in their superannuation and other assets to get them through the rest of their life after their mid-60s, but they are now finding that they are financially stressed. This stress, of course, can cause health strain, whether it be physical or emotional. The cost of living continues to climb each year and the COVID-19 pandemic has highlighted how quickly financial stress can appear to disrupt what appeared to be a 'comfortable' lifestyle for so many.

I hope you can see the logic of my tip. By ensuring that you have good financial planning from a younger age you can ensure that you have the resources available to enjoy your later years from both an active and productive point of view.

> ## TIP
>
> It is never too late to start to get financial advice to assist with your 'retirement' planning. So find a good financial planner (word of mouth or your bank is a good place to start) and start sectioning off some of your income for your retirement investments.

#86 Pick your battles

Inevitably through life you will encounter conflict situations. Depending on how you deal with these situations, you can find a quick resolution and move on, or you can make the situation worse and create chronic long-term stress that affects you far more than you want. Sometimes it is difficult to move away from your principles and values when trying to defend a position, but inevitably on occasions you will find you are dealing with someone who has a completely opposite view — and who can be just as forthright and stubborn in their position. Often these individuals just seek conflict in so many aspects of their life.

In these situations, you can get caught up in unnecessary, time-consuming confrontation that really can serve no long-term gain for yourself, particularly when the issue is a matter of personal perspective. On many occasions, continuing the conflict with the individual is not worth the emotional and physical strain — especially over matters that aren't important in the overall scale of life.

One of the characteristics I hope you develop with experience is to know when to pick your battles. Knowing how to recognise when an individual is quite fixed in their ideas and not prepared to discuss or negotiate their position is one of the best lessons you can learn. In these situations, it is best to remove yourself from the situation and move on to more important things in life. Allowing yourself to stew or dwell on the matter creates negative emotions and has an adverse impact on your overall health and wellbeing. After all, it's only someone's opinion, not legislation. And yes, they may be wrong, but you won't change their perspective.

So, you need to develop a positive attitude to these situations. Is it worth the hassle of continuing a conflict or battle that really serves no purpose in the long term? Move on and allow yourself the freedom of not being held down by the negative attitudes of other people.

While they may feel they have achieved some form of moral or other victory over you in that situation, at least you can rest easy knowing that you are not going to be carrying the negative emotions of the ongoing conflict.

MINDSET

This is another important step in protecting your overall health situation as you move forward. You will definitely sleep better once you master this approach.

#87 Learn to adapt

No matter what stage of life you are in, you'll likely come up against challenges that require you to adapt.

I've mentioned in various points through this book my background in running. The point I'd like to highlight here is that I thought I would run forever. Sadly, that wasn't the case.

I'd grown up running. Since the age of three, I'd competed against my brother in the backyard at our small rural Moolap farm. I then started competitive athletics at age six at the local Little Athletics centre in Geelong. Running was in my DNA. Running soon became part of my life, not only from a competitive point of view but also for the social engagement, fitness and the subsequent opportunity to travel the world. By the time I was in my early 20s, I was competing on the international circuit.

I understood that my ability to deliver elite performances would decline and my competitive career would finish once my medical commitments ramped up and required much more of my time. (I was right about that!) However, I always believed that, regardless of age, I would always run in some capacity. I thought running would continue to be part of my life, both from a fitness point of view, and as an outlet for stress.

Unfortunately, things changed dramatically in 2018 when I developed a permanent knee condition associated with the failure of the protective cushioning cartilage in my kneecap joint. While this is a common affliction of runners, I really had been very lucky throughout my running career. I had not experienced all that many interruptions to my running due to an injury. I'd had an Achilles tendon problem in 1982 that derailed my Commonwealth Games preparation for Brisbane but, before then, a plantar fascia (foot arch) rupture and patellar tendinopathy surgeries were my 'highlight' injuries. Unfortunately, I needed a knee arthroscope surgery in mid-2018 after developing pain that had stopped me while out on a few runs in the preceding weeks. An MRI scan of the knee did not look promising. Likewise, the news was not good following the arthroscope.

I had a significant wear area on the impact-bearing zone of my lower femur bone, which corresponded to the area where runners need great protection and impact cushioning. The pain associated with running was bearable in some ways. But I knew I would only further damage the knee if I kept up regular running. The athlete in me said 'keep going'. The sports physician yelled 'you're cooked'. I had to accept the sad fact that running was no longer going to be a consistent thing in my life. Very few people understood the impact that news had on me emotionally, including my partner at the time. I was pretty flat mentally.

I had to adapt to a challenge that I'd really thought I would never have to face. It took me a lot of deep thinking to accept that my consistent running days were over.

Walking is now my main cardio/aerobic exercise, but I do blend in occasional small runs of one to two minutes in the course of my 50- to 60-minute aerobic sessions. I have termed the activity 'ralking' — a blend of walking with intervals of running. I also advise this ralking program regularly in my practice when guiding injured patients back to their running program.

In my case, my brain at least gets the impression that it is still running even though I'm not really getting the true running experience I loved previously. Nevertheless, the mental boost I get from this little running episode, together with the benefits associated with increased heart rate and fitness during these interval sessions, have been important in me maintaining some semblance of more intense training. I no longer run the 5 to 10 kilometre distances that were an inherent part of my day-to-day and weekly program for so long. Thoughts of running a fun run with my young boys or finishing another half marathon are long gone.

I have adapted.

Adapting for me has been hard but you must deal with these things. In the scale of life, it is hardly a major event, but certainly for someone who had spent over five decades running consistently, it was a big thing. I've come to grips with it over the last couple of years. But I can't say there wasn't some emotional stress associated with it.

Be prepared to adapt if you must change something in life you enjoy. I hope whatever it is that you do for your best exercise activity is something you can continue to do beyond 90 years of age and into the '100 and beyond' target of this book. Good luck.

#88 Know it's never too early to start — or too late

Much of the information contained in this book is appropriate to apply at any age in your lifespan. I believe you are never too young to learn good nutrition and other healthy practices that can be sustained over a lifetime. Good exercise habits and the ability to wisely choose food types are skills that should be taught to children and young adolescents as soon as possible. In this way, the habits of a lifetime are formed, and the knowledge will remain with you as you progress through higher education, middle age and into your most productive years.

Life is a continuing journey of improvement, but it is also important that you put in place the healthy living practices as soon as possible, preferably in childhood.

> **TIP**
>
> If you are a child or young adolescent reading this book, make sure you pass on this information to your parents and get them on board the health program with you!

Similarly, it is never too *late* in life to start making lifestyle changes that can enhance your remaining years. Regardless of whether you are in middle age or the latter decades of your life, it is important to evaluate your health status and consider any improvements you can make based on the information throughout this book. Why not optimise your latter years to improve the quality and content of your life?

For example, it is never too late to begin a well-designed exercise program, combining an appropriate level of aerobic activity with some simple muscle strengthening and flexibility exercises. Muscles can be trained to improve strength, tone, balance and stability regardless of their age.

Many nursing homes now commonly arrange for a therapist to visit the older residents and provide them with some simple exercises to assist with their core and leg strength. This has shown to have great advantages in preventing falls and maintaining mobility. These

MINDSET

exercises may be as simple as repeatedly moving from sitting on a chair to standing to activate the lower back, core, pelvic and thigh muscles. This is a basic strength routine using body weight to assist with strength gains. Similarly, making some improvements to your nutrition plan in later life can assist with providing the appropriate nutrients to assist with muscle repair and maintain gut microbiome health. This will assist with digestion and nutrient utilisation.

Having regular health check-ups in the latter decades of life is also a critical life habit to adopt to help ensure you get ahead of the curve when it comes to detecting any of the predictable illnesses that may occur. Even if you are in your seventh or eighth decade of life, when you follow the advice provided in this book you can still aim for the healthy 100 and beyond target in your healthspan. By making changes even at this late stage of life you may find you can add a further 10 or 15 quality, healthy years to your lifespan. The relevant data shows Australia has a progressively aging population. According to the Australian Institute of Health and Welfare (AIHW), in 2020 4.2 million Australians were aged 65 or over (or 16 per cent of the population). The AIHW estimates that by 2066, 21 to 23 per cent of Aussies will be over 65.

Hence, looking at healthy lifestyle practices is critical — even if you are at a more advanced stage of your lifespan. If you achieve my target of living healthy to 100 years and beyond, then even at age 60, you have over 40 years ahead of you!

'If it is to be, it is up to me.'

I first became aware of this quote when it was delivered to me by my financial adviser and business manager, Damien Smith, during a heartfelt chat back in 1990. We were discussing business plans and overall life direction and Damien, as was his want at the time, was becoming quite philosophical in terms of guiding me in my business and life direction. I had never heard the quote before, but it has stuck with me since.

While the origin and authorship of the phrase is disputed, the meaning is straightforward. You will face many times in your life when you need to make decisions to progress. While it is extremely useful to seek advice from friends, mentors and others in your life, inevitably certain stages of the decision-making process must be self-motivated and enacted based on your thoughts and intuition. Advice coming from others is always useful but putting that advice into action and getting a result fall firmly in the lap of the individual taking the action.

So, when you want to make a certain change in your life, get all the advice and information you can—and then have the fortitude to make a decision and act.

#89 Keep everything in moderation
....

I'm one who believes that we all need to practise everything in moderation, including moderation!

Making changes in your lifestyle to improve health does require discipline and some degree of self-sacrifice, and this can be demanding. I certainly don't want to be seen as a 'wowser' or member of the Fun Police when it comes to having a good time. My tips in this book are not about preventing you from enjoying yourself. If that was the case, my friends who know me well would have stopped reading long ago, because I would have lost all credibility with them!

While moderation is important in terms of nutrition practices, exercise and social enjoyment, I also believe you need to be reasonable in your approach as to how you go about achieving that goal. Hence, my advice here — everything needs to be in moderation, including moderation itself.

We all have times when we might need a day (or two) away from the more rigid protocols required in relation to healthy living practices. You might have a day when you just have that extra glass of wine or a special treat, which may be sugar laden and carbohydrate rich (which, by the way, does add a pleasant dopamine surge). You may also have times when you just don't do that planned exercise session. Don't beat up on yourself. It is okay to have these days — it is, in fact, quite normal. You don't need to train like an Olympic athlete to have the healthy lifestyle I'm advising.

The simple message is while you need to practise moderation in relation to some of the unhealthy foods, alcohol, sugars and other aspects that may not give the best health return, it's also important to enjoy the journey as you go. So, get to it. Be careful, but certainly practise moderation. Even moderation itself needs to be in moderation!

10
Connection

In this final chapter, I discuss the importance of social connection, friendships and lifestyle behaviours that are so common in the world's longest living healthy populations. One recurring theme in these populations is the role of social integration and the happy mindset that comes from this connectivity. I include some of the important ways I believe you can achieve this connectivity in our local area.

I hope you identify with them — there are some fun ideas here!

The importance of family, friendship and community

Having strong connections with your family, friends and community has so many benefits, both for your mental and physical health. Strong connections can boost your happiness and sense of belonging, reduce stress and help you deal with trauma and loss. Not only that, but strong social connections have been shown to reduce the risk of health problems such as high blood pressure and being overweight.

A good friend might even encourage you to change any unhealthy lifestyle habits, such as eating the wrong foods, drinking too much or exercising too little.

You can make and strengthen your connections in so many ways — potentially starting within your own home and social life. But you can also look beyond this, building your local community and making connections wherever you are, whether that be on holiday, enjoying a hobby or with a workout buddy. In the following sections, I explore all of these options and more.

#90 Get married!

When researching the effect of marriage on our health profile, I was surprised at the number of studies that have been done on this topic. While many of the studies are from the United States, extensive studies have also been completed elsewhere in the world, including Australia. And what's the bottom line from all this study? It is healthier to be married than to be single.

As you might imagine the reasons behind this finding are somewhat complicated and involve many factors. Nevertheless, the research shows that married men live longer than lifelong bachelors or divorced men. And it's not only men who gain benefits from being in a committed partnership or marriage. Studies show that when in a committed relationship any individual, male or female, is more likely to have:

- someone to look out for them on a day-to-day basis

- health insurance

- company, so social isolation is avoided

- a better survival after an illness event.

In essence, married individuals live longer, healthier, happier, more active and sexier lives.

Other interesting studies show that the more educated their female spouse is, the better health enjoyed by the male. Men with a more academically qualified spouse have reduced risk of cardiovascular disease, cancer, diabetes, depression and other illnesses compared to unmarried men or men who are married to women who have had less opportunity for higher education.

Make of that what you will!

In addition, married men have been shown to have less mental health issues and more enjoyment in their retirement years than unmarried men.

When it comes to loss of a partner in a relationship, males cope much worse than females. A male who loses his female partner is more likely to die sooner after the bereavement than a female who loses a male partner. This is believed to be associated with the generalisation that men do not cope well with the emotional loss and are less able to care for themselves from the point of view of cooking, nutrition and other day-to-day functions after losing a supportive wife or partner.

The studies outlined here refer to more traditional heterosexual relationship models. This is where the academic studies have so far focused. In our current more modern era of same-sex marriage and de facto permanent relationships, similar studies are needed to determine if the same benefits apply when you are

CONNECTION

in a happy, stable life-partner relationship, regardless of sex or marriage status.

So far the overwhelming evidence is that, particularly for men, it is healthier to be married than unmarried. The studies also show that both men and women benefit from being in a caring, loving, stable, committed relationship. Even when all these factors are not actively present, being married still has advantages.

Yet another factor in aiming for a longer, healthier life.

#91 Enjoy a healthy sex life

Sexual attraction and sexual activity is a basic reproductive function — but it's also so much more than that. And while many individuals do not have an active sex life, sex is still one of the key components that make up societal behaviour.

Sex, especially when orgasm results, releases the pleasure hormone oxytocin, which promotes a feeling of relaxation, wellbeing and happiness. (Refer to chapter 8 for more on the importance of happy hormones.) And, before you start reminding me, yes, I'm well aware that you don't need company to obtain the oxytocin release. The 'self-service' aisle is always available!

How much sex is normal? While this is a commonly asked question, no simple answer is available because it is highly individual. However, a study of 30 000 Americans over four decades found that sex at least once a week was enough to make people happy.

In those individuals who are in a settled, consensual relationship, the frequency of sex will vary enormously — often dictated by work stress, family pressures, illness, hormone levels or other life events. It certainly helps a lot, though, if the sex drives of both partners are in alignment. For 'highly charged' individuals, the frequency may be three or four times per week (or more). At other times the 'gaps' may be weeks. It will fluctuate a lot. One thing is key — open conversation around sexual needs and goals ensures a stable, satisfying relationship. (Oh, and did I mention the self-service aisle for those who choose to add that option?!)

If you're male, you likely will also be pleased to learn that scientific evidence suggests more ejaculations and orgasms lead to lower rates of prostate cancer.

Regardless of your gender, sex can provide the following benefits:

- lower blood pressure

- better immune system

- better heart health, possibly including lower risk for heart disease

- improved self-esteem

- decreased depression and anxiety (dopamine, serotonin release)

- increased libido

- immediate, natural pain relief (endorphin release)

- better sleep

- improved connection with spouse/relationship partner.

In our modern society, sexual behaviour is now accepted as coming in many shapes and sizes. The traditional heterosexual model of

CONNECTION

sexual relationships is still dominant, but same-sex relationships are now much more visible and common, as is sexual identification in relation to bisexuality, monogamy and 'open relationships'.

Some individuals also identify as 'asexual', and sex does not feature as a key component in their social life requirements. I truly believe we are in an era of 'each to your own' — you do not have to comply with traditional models as long as no harm (or illegal activity) is involved.

And what about the benefits of not having sex? In the interests of literary balance, I thought I could add this! Abstinence can be a way to avoid the risks that come with sex — such as pregnancy and STDs. Abstaining from (or avoiding) sex may also help you focus on other things in your life that are important to you, such as friends, sports, activities, education and planning for your future. However, I personally don't think regular consensual, healthy sex interferes with pursuing these goals! Just my humble opinion.

For most, sex is part of our lives, and is a behaviour that contributes to the overall balance of life enjoyment and the pursuit of a longer, healthier active life. The choice is yours on this one!

Eunuchs live longer!

Now here is a piece of health research that is going to make most men shudder. In recent years, several scientific studies have shown that eunuchs—castrated men—can live 15 to 20 years longer than other men. This suggests that the male androgenic hormones play a role in determining the length of your life.

You might ask, 'How do we know this?' and 'Why do we need to know this?' It seems some curious scientists in Korea looked at the historical records of eunuchs who were popular in the Korean imperial court system during the early dynasties as far back as the 14th century, but also reaching through to the early 20th century. By studying the historical records, researchers established that young males who were castrated as boys, but lived an otherwise similar lifestyle in terms of nutrition, environment and social interactivity, lived significantly longer than men who were not castrated in that historical era. Some of these eunuchs lived to an average age of 70, when even the most privileged of males rarely made it past the age of 50. In fact, three examples were even discovered of eunuchs living to the age of 100, which was simply an unheard of age or lifespan in that society.

While the evidence is not completely validated as to the reasons behind this strange phenomenon of men losing their testicles and then living a longer life (that's me shuddering about now!), it is presumably related in some way to the production of male hormones, in particular testosterone. No testicles = no testosterone. (That's me shuddering again!)

More support has been given to this theory by studies that looked at the lifespan of sex offender prisoners who were castrated as part of their punishment. These men lived on average an additional 14 years more than their non-castrated fellow prisoners.

#92 Instil healthy habits in your children

I discuss the role of knowing your family history in helping to predict potential illness conditions at various points through this book. I now want to address the importance of family upbringing as being a separate predictor and influence in health and lifestyle. Unfortunately, if you grow up in a household where your parents set bad lifestyle examples, you are more likely to follow in their footsteps and make the same bad choices.

Studies have shown that if you are exposed at a young age to parents who smoke, do no exercise, have poor nutrition habits or exhibit other high-risk activities (such as drug use), you are at greater risk of being negatively influenced by what you see.

On the other hand, if you grow up in a household with good lifestyle habits, such as healthy nutrition, good exercise and a positive attitude to looking after one's health, you are more likely to adapt these same principles and be healthier. I remain hopeful that young individuals growing up in a household where the examples provided may not be ideal are still able to overcome their environment through their own insight and understanding of the importance of looking after themselves. Nonetheless, it is certainly helpful to have had a good environment and provide a good example in your own household.

If you are a parent, you are responsible for setting a good example for your children in the hope that they will adapt the same principles. While you no doubt focus on setting up your children through good education and financial security in the future, it is equally important that you also invest in their future by providing good examples of healthy behaviours in your own life so that your children (and their children) will be influenced in a positive way. Surely this is one of the greatest legacies we can leave our children and families.

In my own children's schooling, I was impressed by some of the healthy lifestyle lessons that were taught as part of their curriculum. Sometimes they even educated me about some new issues! So these lessons contributed not only to their future wellbeing, but also to me adopting these habits myself. Indeed, the younger generation often has the ability to influence their own parents and grandparents to make changes to provide a healthy lifestyle going forward.

This kind of back and forth certainly contributes to the generational family unit being able to spend a lot more time together in a healthy environment in future years. So, it becomes a two-way street where the parents can influence the children and the children can also influence the parents — what a great combination.

Blue zones and *ikigai*

The regions in the world that have the healthiest, longest living communities have been dubbed the 'blue zones'. The best-known of these zones are Sardinia (Italy), Okinawa Island (Japan), Nicoya Peninsula (Costa Rica), Ikaria (Greece) and Loma Linda (California). These regions are famous for having more inhabitants per capita living healthy lives beyond 100 years than anywhere else on the globe.

One of the most famous is the island off Japan called Okinawa, where it has been documented that the women in particular live long, healthy and productive lives. In fact, the inhabitants of this island in the south of Japan on average live longer than people anywhere else, with many reaching well over 100 years of age.

The challenge, of course, is to understand why this island and other blue zones have such healthy long-living populations — what is their secret? In Okinawa, the inhabitants have a healthy diet, a simple life outdoors in beautiful weather and a high consumption of green tea. However, a lot of the credit to their longevity is also given to the concept of *ikigai*.

CONNECTION

(continued)

The Japanese *ikigai* translates as 'a reason for being'—it is something (or someone) that provides a sense of purpose. It could also translate as the 'happiness of always being busy'. Studies of Ogimi in particular, a village in Okinawa, have revealed that the inhabitants feel a real sense of community involvement and social integration, and this contributes to their happy lifestyle. They have an active social life, help each other out with their day-to-day activities and have a very positive outlook on life. They grow much of their own produce and help in community gardens. Their physical activity levels are above average. In other words, they have *ikigai*, and this has been credited for this happy outlook. As a result, the island of Okinawa has nearly 25 people over the age of 100 for every 100 000 inhabitants. This is way above the average for any other part of the world, except for the other well-performing blue zones.

The concept of retirement, which so often results in people losing their motivation to do things in life, is almost unknown in the blue zones, including Okinawa. In fact, the Japanese language has no word equivalent to 'retirement' in the sense of 'leaving the workforce for good'. The idea that once you retire you cease to do anything and no longer follow your passions is not looked on favourably at all. That's impressive!

Social isolation in Okinawa is almost unheard of. All ages mix together, and generations support each other. Their enthusiasm for life and interaction is infectious (in a healthy way!). Retirement homes are not a flourishing industry! The locals describe themselves as being happy as a result of their social connectivity.

I think the message is extremely clear. If you have a purpose in life, regardless of age, your motivation is increased, and you look forward to each day. If you combine this with healthy living, a good environment, regular activity and community involvement, then I see no reason why we can't reproduce the positive outcomes from the blue zones in other parts of the world.

You need to create your own *ikigai* environment. In some ways, it is such a simple concept to get right. In other ways, the challenges of modern living—with technology, processed foods, busy lifestyles, screen time and online communication rather than face-to-face contact—all result in a society far removed from the blue zones concept. We all need to learn the lessons from these healthy aging individuals and 'strive to thrive' as they clearly do.

I'm not suggesting you relocate to another country in order to achieve your healthy longevity and healthspan. (Although certainly Sardinia appeals to me! They also regularly consume a particular red wine there made from the grenache grape that I enjoy.) Nevertheless, you can look at the lifestyle and environmental factors that lead to such healthy aging and see which elements can be applied to your current location and environment. In this way, you can aim to achieve your own little 'blue zone' in your neighbourhood and community.

This is yet another important step in the healthy aging process and heading towards your target of 100 healthy years and beyond.

#93 Keep in mind that laughter really is medicinal

No doubt you've heard the phrase 'laughter is the best medicine'. The use of humour to lighten a situation and put a smile on someone's face has been used in society for centuries. I remember as a youngster always looking forward to my mother receiving her subscription copy of the *Reader's Digest* magazine, which had a section devoted to jokes. (This section even came under the heading 'Laughter is the best medicine'.) While I was probably too young initially to appreciate or understand some of the jokes printed, I remember many of them putting a smile on my face. I recall even the corny ones made me smile, despite thinking they were quite childish at times — that's humour.

However, with all the studies that highlight the neurochemical benefits of activities we enjoy, it now makes sense that something as pleasurable and simple as laughter would also contribute to the release of happy chemicals such as dopamine and serotonin — the 'feel-good hormones' (refer to chapter 8). In addition, when you're going through some tough times from an emotional point of view, the ability to have a good laugh with a friend or colleague can be soothing and relaxing. It is no coincidence that comedy shows — whether live or in electronic format (theatre, TV series, movies) — are popular with so many audiences wanting some relaxing entertainment. Famous comedy series such as *Seinfeld, Frasier, Cheers* and *Friends* were likely part of your entertainment fabric growing up.

TIP

Keep a sense of humour in your life and take the opportunity to enjoy a good laugh, no matter what other distractions may be happening.

I am not advocating that you make light of a serious situation with comedy, but simply that laughter can be medicinal in terms of helping you live a more calm and enjoyable life. Not all of us can be comedians, but certainly it is useful to be able to watch some of the best in action to put a smile on our face, at least as a short-term distraction. Keep smiling!

#94 Take advantage of the benefits of drinking wine

Now this is perhaps the section that my friends have been looking forward to reading the most. Those who know me well will attest that I am partial to sharing an occasional glass of wine with friends, and this has been a pastime of mine for many years. While an obvious social benefit comes from sharing wine with friends and others, it is really the established health benefits of drinking wine that I wish to address. No, I am actually being serious here!

Wine has been a feature of the human diet for as long as history has been recorded. I take inspiration from the fact that wine was mentioned on so many occasions in the Bible! Surely, if it was good enough for Jesus and the Apostles at the last supper, there must be a justification for having it in my own life!?

But, in all seriousness, wine has existed since the origins of food production and farming, which emerged approximately 10000 years ago. Fresh produce deteriorated very quickly, but our early ancestors observed that the process of fermentation of these fruits and vegetables did preserve them for a longer period of time, even in the absence of cold storage. History records that many beverages consumed in that era originated from fermented vegetables, cereals, fruits and even honey from beehives.

Fortunately, some clever individuals determined that grape fermentation was also possible, and this led to the concept of exploring ways of producing various types of wine. The initial motivation for

CONNECTION

producing wine was purely from a social consumption point of view, with the end game generally being intoxication. While I would argue that this is still a very common practice or motivation for some in the consumption of wine, we now have far more evidence that a huge range of health benefits are also associated with the moderate consumption of wine, particularly red wine.

A brief history of wine

History documents that the earliest evidence of wine production is from the areas around Georgia (6000 BCE), Persia (5000 BCE) and Italy (4000 BCE). The Spaniards did not want to be left out and also managed to get onto this newfound social activity around the same time as the Italians. In France, Christian monks have been credited with establishing France's reputation as one of the best winemaking countries in the world. Once again, there is a religious component to this message of the health benefits of wine.

Agreement has not been reached as to whether one individual can be credited with inventing wine. In Greek mythology, Dionysus, the son of Zeus, has been credited with inventing wine when living on Mount Nysa (surrounded by mountain nymphs). This is one of the reasons Dionysus is often referred to as the God of Wine.

However, my favourite story relates to a Persian princess who found herself out of favour with the King of Persia. She tried to commit suicide by drinking from a jar of rotting grapes but, rather than dying, began to feel better and a lot happier after drinking the fermented fruit. Eventually she passed out from intoxication, but when she woke up the king had decided that he liked her new social attitude and readmitted her to the kingdom in a privileged position.

I am not sure we can apply this scenario to too many modern social occasions, but I suspect a similar scenario has played out on several occasions where a night 'on the grapes' has resulted in the establishment (or re-establishment) of a relationship!

Red wine—the healthier option?

While many different varieties of both white and red wine (as well as other combinations) are available, the major research on wine relates to red wine being the healthiest option. It is important to note I am referring here to wine enjoyed in moderation, rather than the huge over-consumption that some individuals might pursue. Moderation with respect to wine usually means one to three glasses in a sitting, depending on body size and the type of wine consumed.

The reasons red wine is healthier include the following:

- *Improvements in gut health:* Red wine is antibacterial and was used in the past to treat stomach irritation and other digestive disorders.

- *Rich in antioxidants:* Grapes contain potent antioxidants that are beneficial in reducing metabolic damage done by normal body oxidation processes. The skin of grapes is particularly rich in antioxidant compounds called 'polyphenols'. (Red wines are fermented with the grape skins and seeds while white wines are not.) The antioxidant resveratrol is a polyphenol that has been shown to be intrinsically beneficial in assisting repair of damaged body cells from free radical metabolic reactions. Polyphenols have been linked to the reduction in diseases such as cardiac disease, diabetes, Alzheimer's and Parkinson's.

CONNECTION

- *Reduction in inflammation:* As just mentioned, red wine is rich in the extremely important compound resveratrol. Resveratrol is also a potent anti-inflammatory agent, and it is well known that inflammation can cause a number of significant illnesses in the body. Inflammation can be brought about through poor diet, minimal exercise and increased stress. All these contribute to increased risk of cardiac disease, autoimmune problems and the potential onset or aggravation of cancer processes. The aging process is clearly accelerated as a result of these illnesses. The value of resveratrol in wine is probably equal to or more important than the antioxidant value of wine.

- *Regulation of blood glucose (sugars):* Resveratrol is also capable of assisting with blood sugar control in normal people as well as people with diabetes. It has been shown to be beneficial for lowering blood fats (cholesterol) and even helping with blood pressure management. These benefits obviously contribute to a reduced risk of the two main causes of death — heart disease and stroke.

- *Antidepressant function:* Drinking moderate amounts of wine each day (note the word moderate) has been shown to reduce depression in middle-aged adults. Now, you may say that if you drink enough wine, you will be unlikely to feel depressed about anything in the world, but this is not the point of my discussion of its antidepressant role!

Vintages and varietals

I have already made the point that red wine is a healthier option than white wine. Of course, both are enjoyable in social circumstances, but if we are really being specific about the health benefits of wine drinking, then red certainly is the number one choice. Not all red wines are equal when it comes to health benefits, however. The concentration of antioxidants and resveratrol in red wine can depend on the type of red wine grape used and the winemaking process.

Studies have shown that grapes that undergo the most 'stress' during their ripening process also produce the greatest defence for themselves, and so contain more of the important chemicals that are associated with survival and health. For example, pinot noir is a difficult grape to grow compared to some of the other red wine varieties, such as cabernet sauvignon, shiraz, merlot and grenache. While all of these varieties contain health benefits, the pinot noir variety provides the most, due to the stress it undergoes during its life cycle. It produces a higher concentration of resveratrol, the important health compound. In Sardinia, one of the blue zones of the world and known for its healthy longevity, the preferred wine is a local grenache.

As my friends might imagine, I have been sampling these health-producing wine varieties in the name of medical research in recent years.

By the way, the higher health benefits are also true of fruits and vegetables that are grown naturally and undergo some degree of stress during their ripening. Naturally grown organic fruit and vegetables do tend to have a higher nutrient value than the 'privileged' hot house grown varieties, which grow in a protected environment and are not exposed to the stress of weather, birds or other attacks. Organically grown produce need to mount a defence for their own survival, and this process again increases their antioxidants. Similarly, the use of pesticides and other products is not helpful if you are trying to get the highest nutrient health value from fruit and vegetables.

In many other parts of this book, I have advocated for the important role of regular physical activity and healthy nutrition in providing so many of the health benefits that can lead to a long, healthy life. Red wine can be safely added to the list of lifestyle choices, provided you follow my rules regarding moderation! So, next time you are out enjoying a glass or two of wine with friends, you can happily tell them you are contributing to your health status — under my guidance!

#95 Have a hobby

Many of the hours in your typical week are likely taken up with work, and personal and family activities. You might often feel like you are left with very little time for other pursuits. However, by adopting a hobby — whether it be gardening, painting or a book club — you're giving yourself an opportunity for some stimulation independent of your normal weekly activities. You're often also adding an opportunity for some social connectivity with others who have the same hobby or interests as you.

While a hobby may be an individual pursuit that you do in isolation, it also may involve being involved with a community charity group, suburban walks looking at historical sites, or even helping with a local junior sports club, even if you don't have children participating in that sport. These hobby activities contribute to an overall harmony in your week and give you another dimension of achieving that illusive mix of compulsory commitments and optional choices in your structured life pursuits.

You have so many different options for what your hobby could be — the list is almost endless. Some people choose a hobby that is quite dynamic such as hiking, bushwalking, sailing or rock climbing. Others might choose more passive hobbies such as painting, collecting or reading. In some ways, the choice is irrelevant because it is not so much whether you are physically active during the hobby time that is important here, but whether you have something that is emotionally challenging and satisfying.

Having a pleasurable hobby will also help with increasing your daily DOSE of happy hormones (refer to chapter 8). Looking forward to doing these activities, whether you do them after hours or on weekends, only adds to the positive emotions connected to having some enjoyable time away from your formal commitments.

The benefits of your hobby are often multi-layered. For example, when you join a book club or a community gardening project, you not only benefit from the hobby itself (fresh vegetables anyone?), but you're also able to interact with other people. I've noted elsewhere that social interaction has been shown to be an important part of the anti-aging process and part of maintaining good physical and emotional health. I have a long-term patient who is well into his 80s. I have looked after his bad knees for many years and one of the benefits for him is his ongoing ability to contribute to his community produce garden — and I get the benefits of fresh zucchini, squash and tomatoes (all organic)!

The concept of social interaction and social connectivity is a common thread in so many of the studies performed on those communities around the world where health and longevity beyond 100 years are common. (Refer to the breakout box 'Blue zones and *ikigai*', earlier in this chapter.) It doesn't really matter what your hobby is — if you do it with other people, a critical benefit is the social engagement that is associated with the hobby group as much as the activity itself.

In my earlier days, I would have listed one of my hobbies as collecting red wine! While I may have had an ulterior motive to that pastime initially, I am now much more aware that red wine is actually a 'health supplement' when taken in moderation and at appropriate times. (Refer to the previous section for more on this.) While my wine collecting is less aggressive these days than it was in the past (my budget has been reduced!), I am still recommending that it is important to have other pursuits that you would consider as a hobby, such as those I've included here.

So, get to it — check in your local community for hobby opportunities. The local council is a good place to start. A community Facebook page usually provides a wealth of information also.

#96 Listen to whatever is music to your ears

Surely music would qualify as one of the most pleasant and enjoyable ways to spend our downtime. Music has been used as a form of therapy for many years in psychology, and can assist people with anxiety and depression. But even in the simplest scenario, it is one of the more pleasurable things to do at the end of a busy day.

I find nothing is better than sitting down with a relaxing glass of wine, putting on some of my favourite music and just enjoying the experience. You might even have your favourite playlist ready and loaded on your mobile device. It doesn't really matter what your taste in music is — you might prefer calming, classical or acoustic ballad music, or you might find listening to heavy metal or hard rock music relaxing. Whatever floats your boat is the choice for you to make.

Studies have shown listening to music also releases some of the 'happy hormones' discussed in chapter 8. Because music can be soothing and calming, it has a relaxing effect and has been associated with the release of certain neurochemicals, including dopamine and serotonin.

So, while most people will consider music a form of entertainment, be aware that it can also be a form of therapy and relaxation that contributes to your wellbeing, particularly from an emotional and mental point of view.

> **TIP**
>
> Creating a playlist of your own favourite choices is a lot of fun. You can then use that playlist as a form of distraction when you are out doing your exercise session, be it walking, running or even gardening. Even lying on the beach or by the pool lends itself to some background chill-out music for me.

The challenge is there for you now — create a favourites playlist (or several) that will give you some relaxation time and add to your wellbeing.

Happy humming!

#97 Plan a holiday

Who doesn't like the opportunity to take a break from their normal routine and 'get away from it all'? Most commonly, this takes the form of a vacation or holiday where you get a chance to travel to a different location and change your routine, hopefully in a more relaxed and beneficial way.

Taking a holiday in a pleasurable environment (with good company) is a sure way of getting your daily DOSE of happy hormones. Apart from the physical recovery that may occur from having a less-structured routine of work hours and physical work stress, you can also gain the benefit of being in an environment where you have

CONNECTION

more time to undertake a regular exercise routine on a daily basis. The added value of being outside and getting sunshine and vitamin D adds to your health boost. (I personally prefer a warm summer environment for a holiday, although of course others choose a challenging vacation, which may include hiking, mountain climbing or travelling to the snow.)

Holidays may also give you the opportunity to catch up with friends, which then contributes to your social interaction and connectivity. If you have a partner and/or children, holidays also allow for family time and building these connections. You can build valuable memories for the future and reconnect with the important things in life.

The anticipation of looking forward to a well-planned holiday can also be a pleasurable stimulus. With modern life being as busy as it is these days, it is usually necessary to plan ahead for these holidays, making sure you include opportunities to restore and recover from both a physical and emotional standpoint. This gives you something to look forward to, and a target to work towards. I know I have become much better at planning breaks from my busy work routine on a more regular basis now than I did in the past.

TIP

You likely need to plan your holiday time around work leave, school holidays and your preferred seasonal weather. But also keep in mind that this break can be as short as a long weekend away. You'll still gain the benefits from getting away to a different location, reducing your stress and building connections.

So, where is your next 'holiday for health' going to be?

#98 Enjoy the perfect holiday
.... with the seven Ss

This topic had its origins at a rowdy dinner party discussion among close friends many years ago. We were discussing what components made the complete or perfect holiday experience. I offered that I had condensed my requirements down to the 'seven Ss'. This resulted in the conversation becoming even more lively and extending for a much longer period of time!

Naturally, we had a few giggles as people tried to come up with what my components were. Over the subsequent years, I have discussed this topic on many occasions and, in fact, the original 'seven Ss' list has been supplemented by the ideas of many of my friends over conversations and dinner parties since.

In the previous section, I discuss the importance of planning regular holidays. Holidays certainly allow you to look forward to a relaxing future event and refresh both physically and mentally in your time away. The choices of location can be quite variable, but ultimately you will look for new experiences or places that meet your requirements.

To help you with your planning and decision-making, I outline here the 'seven Ss' that I believe combine to make the perfect holiday.

Sleep

Despite the many predictable cheeky suggestions from others, sleep has always been my number one component. I discuss the value of sleep in chapter 8, emphasising its important role in refreshing the mind and body. In our busy lives we are often skimping on the amount of optimal sleep we get, and this ultimately has a draining effect on our overall performance in life.

CONNECTION

The opportunity to go on vacation and not have to worry about an early morning alarm clock is one of the joys of my holiday planning. That doesn't mean that I may not still rise early in the morning to do a beautiful fitness walk in a national park or along a coastline or beach. But the simple ability (and treat) of allowing the body to get the amount of sleep it needs rather than being locked into a strict routine related to work, meetings, peak hour travel or other commitments is so important. A good bed, good pillow and good sleep environment are a critical part of holiday time, and sleep remains number one on my list of perfect holiday requirements.

Sunshine

No doubt you have your preferences for your ideal environment for a holiday. In my case, I have always drifted towards preferring a holiday in a warm environment where I can take in sunshine and outdoor activities most conveniently. And, as discussed in chapter 8, enjoying the sun (safely) is so important for topping up your vitamin D and improving mood.

In Australia, we are lucky to have so many holiday locations that have warm weather and potentially a beach or ocean-side location. We also have the ability to travel to our neighbouring countries closer to the equator where the weather is predictably warm and sunny. Australia has so many wonderful choices, but I have also enjoyed holidays in Hawaii, Thailand, Fiji, Vietnam, Bali, Langkawi, Singapore, and other easily accessible destinations. Of course, further afield you can also travel in the Northern Hemisphere summer to wonderful locations around the Mediterranean or perhaps the Caribbean. The choices are endless, and perhaps you prefer something different, but for me the option to spend time outdoors, both relaxing and exercising, as well as getting my vitamin D sunshine dose, is one of the enjoyable parts of a perfect holiday

Seafood

Eating well and from healthy choices on my holiday is a priority. I enjoy seafood, and healthy omega-3 rich fish and other seafood choices are a great source of protein and nutrition. Choosing a holiday venue close to the ocean, where there is usually an abundance of fresh seafood available on menus, helps make this option easily accessible. Seafood always goes well with healthy salads, so I feel like I am making an effort on my holidays to really keep a good approach with my nutrition plan.

Sweating

This is the part where my exercise routine and workouts kick in. The sweating I am referring to here does not include sitting around a hot pool baking in the sun or spending time in a sauna. What I'm talking about is getting out and doing some of the cardio aerobic exercise that is so important to our health. In the past, I used to love exploring my holiday destinations by going out for a lengthy run, but these days I have adapted to a mixture of exercise walking with some occasional intermittent slow runs ('ralking'). It doesn't matter what exercise you choose — it can by cycling, swimming, walking, a gym fitness session, perhaps some yoga or Pilates. The point is holidays are a great time to have a consistent exercise routine.

On holidays, I usually prefer to get my exercise session done early in the day, particularly if I am in a pleasant hot environment, but sometimes it can be done in the early evening prior to the dinner meal. The advantage of getting it out of the way early is that you can relax through the remainder of the day and head for those late afternoon sunset drinks that are so often on offer at the holiday resorts! Bring on 'happy hour'!

So, when planning your next holiday, make sure you have a good opportunity to work up a sweat.

Sipping

This is where you get to be a bit inventive and have some fun. My sipping relates to my drinking habits when I am away on holidays, and this is usually part of the fun of catching up with your partner and other close friends who may be with you. With summer lunches, I tend to avoid red wines, so my go-to sipping beverage (if alcohol) has been soave, chablis or pinot grigio. Champagne will always get a look-in depending on the day and location, and sometimes in the evening a lightly chilled pinot noir is just the thing.

If you don't drink alcohol, you can look for some of the great non-alcoholic options available, including mocktails, non-alcohol beers or other refreshing beverages to make sure that you enjoy the sipping component of your holiday. However, always remember to drink lots of chilled water as part of the process to keep yourself well hydrated regardless of any of your other sipping treats.

Social reading

Part of the enjoyment for me of being on holidays is doing some relaxed reading. In my normal working life, I do heaps of reading, but it is mainly related to new medical information, websites, sports medicine updates, journals, and other health-related material (including research for this book). Being away on holidays is an opportunity to catch up on some reading material that doesn't relate specifically to my working life.

I am fortunate to live near one of Melbourne's most famous and awarded bookshops as well as belonging to a number of online book purchasing websites. During the year, I tend to accumulate several books that I put aside to read, and these are usually designated as my 'holiday reading'. Of course, I try to get some reading done during the normal year as a break from the more formal work-related reading, but far more often these books become my reading material during travel and holiday time. I also own a Kindle reader that I have found extremely useful for travel. However, for me nothing beats the sensation and tactile experience of having a printed book in my hand. I like to make notes in the margin of many of the books or highlight important sections. It has been a habit of mine for many years. In fact, it is unusual to find me reading any sort of material without a pen in my hand (even the daily newspaper).

Holidays provide the opportunity to give your brain a break from the more formal workday reading materials and take in some novels or other material such as travel or wine information books. So keep note of your favourite topics or authors, and take them away with you.

Sex

Yes, of course you were expecting sex to be in the seven Ss! It might come as no surprise to you that many will put this up as the first S when we have our discussions about the seven Ss. I have regularly had to reassure all and sundry who are listening that sleep is definitely number one on my personal list. Nevertheless, regular physical intimacy can be hard to achieve during our busy working lives. Long working days, fatigue, family and children commitments and a whole host of other issues can interfere with opportunity for you and your partner to enjoy regular personal time.

Being away on holidays can provide the opportunity for less pressure and more time for quality one-on-one time with your partner. The opportunity for more sleep-ins or perhaps early nights in bed provides an environment that is not always easy to achieve back at home in the normal busy weeks. There is something about sun, seafood, sipping and the holiday environment that can lead to a more relaxed approach to personal time together — both in you and in your partner.

Sometimes, it is even important to plan an afternoon nap on holidays to give you both a chance to refresh and spend some personal time together. (I suggest 3.30 pm to 5 pm can be a very important time slot during the holiday schedule!) So, I understand that sex may not be in the top seven Ss for everyone, but given how often it has appeared in the conversations when discussing this topic, it does rank in my top seven.

Supplementary Ss

Many supplementary Ss have been suggested over the years by my close friends. The list continues to expand, and I am sure you will be able to add your own important Ss to the list after giving some consideration to this concept. I look forward to hearing from many of you as to the suggestions.

Here are some further Ss that have been suggested over the years:

+ *Swimming:* This can be your regular holiday physical activity pursuit, particularly if your holiday is near a beach or resort with pool. It certainly forms part of the 'sweat' component.

+ *Surf:* This could be riding surf boards, but could also include stand up paddle boards or boogie boards, or simply body surfing. You do need to be more confident with the ocean and waves and have good swimming skills.

+ *Sand:* Walking along the sand or lying on the sand reading a good book can be relaxing (although the downside can be getting covered in sand or having sand in your swimsuit!).

+ *Snow:* We are lucky in Australia that many of us have snow resorts in a reasonably accessible travel time from our homes. Snow holidays do require a little bit more organisation and a larger wardrobe choice, and come with many add-on expenses such as lessons and lift passes. Nevertheless, they can be a fantastic enjoyable family holiday.

+ *Shopping:* Again, if you are busy in your normal working life, you may not have time to do regular shopping that you would like to do, particularly for personal items such as clothing. Bringing home an item from a trip is always a great memory and, of course, you may have time during your 'sweat' walking activities to visit some of the local markets or shopping centres.

+ *Sounds:* Soothing sounds such as the sound of waves, the rainforest or some other relaxing ambient noise can be a great source of relaxation at night and can help with getting quality sleep.

+ *Sunsets:* One of the joys of being in a beautiful location is taking in the amazing sunsets. These always create a highlight and provide some fantastic photographic opportunities for memories of your holidays.

+ *Sightseeing:* Whether you're visiting a foreign country or simply a different part of your own country, getting out and about to create memories, take some photographs and visit some of the important historical locations or beautiful natural vistas can be a highlight for your holiday memories.

+ *Socialising:* If you enjoy socialising, the opportunity to meet new friends (or spend more time with your home-

(continued)

based friends that you don't see all that often) is an advantage provided by holiday time away, particularly if you are staying in a large resort or popular destination. I have met many people on holidays who have become lifelong friends.

+ *Solitude:* In contrast to the preceding point, you may like the peace and quiet of being alone on your holidays. You can take the opportunity to get some quiet personal time to relax, exercise and perhaps catch up with that important social reading.

+ *Serenity:* Similar to the last point, a holiday—especially if you choose a secluded location—can give you the opportunity to have some peaceful quiet time away from the hustle and bustle associated with your home-based busy lifestyle.

+ *Silence:* This might be a little harder to achieve, depending on the location of your holiday, but is a similar theme to the serenity and solitude just discussed. Again, this is an individual choice but it can be incorporated into a part of your day regardless of the location.

What Ss do you have to add to my list? Let me know!

#99 Have a workout buddy

Committing to a regular workout session can be challenging. One of the greatest ways to ensure better compliance is to arrange to do the activity with a buddy—this could be a friend, work colleague or neighbour. By making a commitment to meet up at a certain time or certain spot each day, you have given yourself more motivation to actually turn up—because you don't want to let the other person down. If you're thinking about not turning up, particularly for an early morning session, the mild 'guilt trip' can be enough to get you up and going!

Many people are very enthusiastic at the start of their exercise program, with great intentions about what they want to achieve. Unfortunately, this enthusiasm can drop away very quickly if the exercise sessions are not designed in an interesting way, or you do not have a companion to share them with.

Homes and garages are full of unused exercise equipment such as stationary bikes and treadmills, all bought with enthusiasm and the best of intentions. Many become dust and cobweb collectors—or an expensive clothes horse! Gym memberships often go unused after the initial month of frantic use.

> ## TIP
> One of the best things you can do is commit to a regular workout with someone else. This means you are more likely to be compliant with your regular program—and the mutual motivation is a huge bonus also.

#100 Never judge a book by its cover

I cannot recall how old I was when I first encountered this phrase, but I know I was quite young. It has stuck with me since. While the literal meaning was obvious to me, I also understood the context in which it was used. Throughout life, we have all encountered individuals whom we initially assumed or judged to be a certain style of person, only to find that we had completely misread the situation.

CONNECTION

In the literal sense, the term has also been a recurring theme, particularly in my life. For example, on many occasions I have enthusiastically started out on a book based on its title or cover, only to then really struggle to get into the story. On other occasions, books have been recommended to me that I certainly did not think seemed appealing on the surface. However, once I have drilled deeper, the actual content turned out to be riveting and most rewarding to read. (In the case of this book, I hope both the cover and the content appeals to you!)

Similarly, with individuals in your life, understanding what's behind the external veneer is really important. You likely know people who appear to have an extremely well organised external appearance to their lives. They may be well presented, engaging with conversation and appear to have everything going well in their life. When you get to know these people, you will often find that they have many of the same struggles that are associated with life's challenges. They may be experiencing career struggles, financial hardship, relationship issues or, more importantly, maybe suffering from anxiety or other mental health disorder that does not manifest so easily until you get to know them.

It is quite easy to be envious of someone else's life when you see them only from the outside. When you take time to learn more about them, you may discover that, despite their external appearance of apparent success and obvious wealth, their life can actually be quite unhappy and miserable behind the external façade.

In a similar vein, I have known many people who from an external appearance appear to be quite understated and underachieving, but when you do get to know them, you find that they have an extremely successful corporate or business career and have a very harmonious life with things under control. These people have certainly discovered and are optimising their *ikigai* (discussed earlier in this chapter).

I have learnt on many occasions never to judge a patient sitting in my waiting room when I am meeting them for the first time. While some might appear introverted and even sometimes unkempt and scruffy (no names here!), I have often been surprised at how accomplished and articulate these individuals are once you spend some time getting to know them. I have learnt how much these people can teach me in relation to the things they have achieved in their life. The converse is also true. Some people are all 'froth and bubble' on the surface, but shallow beneath.

I think the lesson here is reasonably straightforward. It is important to really get behind the external veneer of someone before judging them. Often you will be surprised at the positives and, unfortunately, at times the negatives will also become evident. Never rush in too quickly—first, take the opportunity to find the real person behind their external presentation. You need to make an effort to explore beyond their 'game face'. It is quite rewarding to make that effort to get to know someone and to really show an interest—they will often return the favour in spades. It does not take a lot of energy to put some time into getting to know someone and showing an interest. It is a great characteristic to develop in your pathway in life, and on your way to 100 and beyond.

CONNECTION

Conclusion: What now?

The 'fountain of youth' doesn't exist. If something similar does exist, you access it through following a healthy lifestyle, and making wise choices to promote anti-aging effects and minimise the health risks of modern life stresses.

The evidence for the health benefits of regular aerobic and cardio activity with a mixture of some strength and flexibility training are now well established in the medical literature. The best health supplement does not come in a bottle, pill or injection, but is associated with some active effort on behalf of the individual — that's you.

Throughout this book, I've provided you with information on ways to pursue healthy living. As a bonus, if you follow these strategies and tips you can achieve extra productivity in what you do and more illness-free years in your life — your 'healthspan' increase.

You don't have to get every single tip right. You can pick and choose, and even small changes can have significant health impacts. You don't have to be perfect — no-one is! But I hope you do something with this information — as Persian poet Saadi wrote way back in 1258,

'Whoever acquires knowledge and does not practise it resembles him who ploughs his land and leaves it unsown.'

I hope you now understand that you have more control over your health destiny than you might have realised. Bad health is not set by fate—much of it is lifestyle related. Maintaining good health is not necessarily a passive entitlement. You have to actively contribute through a combination of lifestyle changes, nutrition and exercise. Many of the risk factors associated with ill health can be identified, and these can then be modified by taking action to correct their negative effects.

It is important to recognise early health warnings so that modifications can be made and tragedies such as late detection of advanced disease, cancers or cardiac deaths can be offset. Many diagnostic tests are now available that can help identify and plan modifications and even reverse the trends of ill health.

It is also important to remember that the greatest health gain comes from changing from doing no regular physical activity to doing something, even if it is as little as 60 minutes a week of walking—or just 15 minutes, four times a week. This can be achieved by most individuals in the context of their busy lives. You can then progressively add to the 60 minutes per week as your exercise program is adopted and customised according to your needs.

The target of living to a healthy 100 and beyond is very realistic—especially if you are still in your middle stages of life. Regardless, it is never too late to improve lifestyle habits. Go for it today!

Some quick tips to leave you with

As you continue on your journey to 100 and beyond, here are some quick reminders and tips to take with you.

My 10 positive reminders for taking charge of your health

1. You have more control over your health destiny than you realise.

2. Most risk factors are identifiable and many can be modified.

3. Good health is not a passive entitlement — *you* have to contribute.

4. The evidence for the health benefits of cardio and strength training are indisputable.

5. Recognising early health warnings can help offset illness onset.

6. The best health supplement doesn't come in a bottle, pill or injection.

7. Testing is available to plan lifestyle modifications and reverse trends in ill health predictors.

8. The biggest health gain comes from changing from nothing to something (60 minutes of exercise per week).

9. Don't expect sudden big gains — set small, achievable targets and the healthy habits will accumulate to create more sustainable long-term benefits.

10. Your greatest reward comes from knowing you are making the changes that can lead to a healthier, happier and longer life.

My top 10 tips for healthy living

1. Don't be overweight (but be active even if you are).

2. Eat a varied, balanced and nutritious diet.

3. Do some regular aerobic and strength activity.

4. Get enough sleep.

5. Learn not to stress over the little things.

6. Have some lifelong friends and mentors.

7. Recognise early health warnings.

8. Get a good GP (or health promotion doctor).

9. Understand that moderation is better than excess.

10. Choose your parents wisely!

My 10 key messages

1. Healthy living is a complex blend of many components.

2. Everyone is individual—responses to different strategies vary.

3. You have more influence and control over your health than you realise.

4. Healthy longevity is not just about good genetics.

5. You're never too old and it's never too late to make healthy lifestyle changes.

6. Proper nutrition is critical and undervalued.

7. Exercise is medicine — and amazing!

8. Your body is your best pharmacy.

9. Health check-ups are essential.

10. Social connectivity is powerful and nurtures healthy longevity.

Index

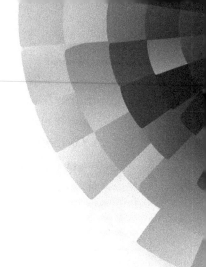

adenosine triphosphate
(ATP) 105, 106
aging process
aim for 100 and beyond 7–8
cellular structures 4–5
death 5–7
healthy lifestyle 8–11
signs of 3–4
AIHW *see* Australian
Institute of Health and
Welfare (AIHW)
alcohol consumption 150–151
alcohol, smoking, obesity,
sedentary and sugar
(ASOSS) 54–55
Alzheimer's disease 42–44
amylase 173
aneurysm 35
anxiety 40
arrhythmia 94
arthroscopic surgery 219

ASOSS *see* alcohol, smoking,
obesity, sedentary and
sugar (ASOSS)
attention to detail
(ATD) 260–261
Australia
cervical cancer in 59
health and illness in 15–17
holiday locations 308
life expectancy in 176
osteoporosis 60
skin cancers 202
stroke events 26
Australian Bureau of Statistics
(ABS) 16, 50
Australian Cancer Council 56
Australian Institute of Health
and Welfare (AIHW) 6,
26, 50, 282
bowel cancer 31–32
breast cancer 36

Australian Institute of Health
and Welfare (AIHW)
(*Continued*)
cancer data 28–29
cervical cancer 59
medicine prescriptions 72–73
osteoporosis 60–61
prostate cancer 56
skin melanoma 201
smoking 200
suicide death, male
vs. female 63
tobacco 199
Australia Stroke
Foundation 26–28

Baird, Anthony 106
basal metabolic rate
(BMR) 81
battles 276–278
behaviour 15, 51
Beyond Blue 65
blood pressure 33–35
blue zones 293–295
bowel cancer 31–33
brain health 41–44
food for 118–122
brain neurotransmitters 82
breast cancer 35–37, 58–59
breathing habit 196–197
built-in audio instruction
system 228
burnout 247–249

caffeine consumption 146–147
calcium storage 107
calories counting, in nutrition
plan 158–160
cancer
bowel 31–33
breast 35–37, 58–59
cervical 59
lung 28–31
prostate 56–58
skin 202
Cancer Australia 29
Cannon, Walter 242
carbohydrates 126–127
cardiac health check-up 70–71
cardio (aerobic) activity 89
cardiopulmonary
resuscitation (CPR) 227
catecholamines 191
cellular health/
breakdown 106–107
Centre for Behavioural
Research in Cancer
(CBRC) 29–30
cervical cancer 59
children
healthy habits in 291–293
mindset 252–254
chocolate, for body
health 133–135
chronic illness medical
conditions
blood pressure 33–35

boosting immunity 46–47

bowel cancer 31–33

brain health 41–44

breast cancer 35–37

education and prevention 23

epigenome protection
44–46

health conditions, in
2021 16–17

heart disease 24–25

lungs protection 28–31

mental health 38–41

stroke 26–28

citric acid cycle 106

coffee, for heart health
143–146

cold water immersion
therapy 223–225

colonoscopy 32

colorectal cancer *see*
bowel cancer

compassion 265–266

*The Complete Book of
Running* (Fixx) 94

connection
family, friends and
community 285–286

healthy habits, in
children 291–293

hobby 302–304

laughter 295–297

marriage 286–288

music 304–305

'never judge a book by its
cover' 315–317

sex life 288–291

vacation/holiday 305–306

wine 297–302

workout 314–315

convenience food 114, 131

Cooper, Kenneth 83

COVID-19 pandemic
financial stress 276

immunity 46, 123

mental health 39

vaccinations 234

Dads In Distress 65

dark chocolate 134

death 5–7

deep-phase sleep 177

defibrillators 227–228

dementia 42

deoxyribonucleic acid
(DNA) 5

epigenome 44–46

depression 40

diabetes 132–133

diastolic blood pressure 33

digestive tract, structure of 115

digital rectal examination
(DRE) 57

DNA *see* deoxyribonucleic
acid

dog, taking for walk 209–211

dopamine 190–192

DOSE hormones 115, 190
  dopamine 190–192
  endorphins 194–195
  oxytocin 192–193
  serotonin 193–194
dreams 187–189

endorphins 82, 194–195
energy production 106
environment 14–15, 51
epigenetics 45
epigenome protection 44–46
exercise
  cardio (aerobic)
    activity 88, 89, 222
  challenge 220–221
  clothing and equipment
    planning 101–102
  components, to improve good
    health 81–83
  description of 79
  excuses 97–99
  flexibility and
    stretching 90–91
  for good health 18–19
  as health supplement 83–84
  important medicine 79–80
  increase walking
    speed 103–104
  lifespan and healthspan
    with 109–111
  medical screening 84–86
  mitochondria 105–108

motivation 92–93
never too early/late 280–282
nicotinamide adenine
  dinucleotide 108–109
recovery, time for 100–101
right exercise program 87–88
small changes, for big
  gains 99–100
strength training 89–90
stress management 246
sudden death during 94–95
10 000 steps per
  day 104–105
time spending for 95–97

faecal occult blood (FOB) test 32
family history 235–237
fasting 161–163
FAST test, for stroke 28
fats, good *vs.* bad 128–129
feel good hormone *see* serotonin
female deaths, in Australia 6–7
ferritin levels, for women's
  health 59–60
financial planning 274–276
FITT principle 91–92
Fixx, Jim 94, 95
food labelling 171–172
fuel consumption, for
  muscles 81

gastrointestinal (GI) tract 114
genetics 14, 51

geroscience 4

glycaemic index 126–127, 130

goal setting 258–260

good bacteria 116–117

good health

 behaviour 15

 environment 14–15

 exercise components, to

  improve 81–83

 genetics 14

 health and illness, in

  Australia 15–17

 health check-up 17

 overview of 13

 physical activity and

  exercise 18–19

gut-brain axis system 115

gut health

 breeding good

  bacteria 116–117

 digestive tract,

  structure of 115

 gut microbiome 115–116

gut microbiome 115–116

habits

 breathing 196–197

 cardio and aerobic

  exercise 222

 cold water immersion

  therapy 223–225

 defibrillators 227–228

 dog for walk 209–211

 exercise challenge 220–221

 family history 235–237

 incidental activity 204–205

 jet lag 228–230

 joint health 212–213

 osteoarthritis pain, treatment

  for 216–220

 parking 208–209

 postcodes 226

 quit smoking 198–201

 seaside view 232–233

 simple changes 175–176

 skin protection 201–204

 sleep *see* sleep

 stairs 207–208

 stand up yourself 205–206

 sunshine 230–232

 vaccinations 233–235

happy hormones *see*

 DOSE hormones

Head to Health 65

health check-up

 age for 68–69, 71–72

 building own

  pharmacy 72–75

 cardiac 70–71

 components, of proper

  69–70

 overview of 67–68

healthspan 10–11

health supplement,

 exercise as 83–84

healthy lifestyle 8–11

healthy living
  messages 322–323
  positive reminders 321
  tips for 322
heart, food for 122–123
heart disease 24–25
heat production 107
high blood pressure 34–35
high intensity interval
  training (HIIT) 92
hobby 302–304
holiday
  planning 305–306
  with 'seven Ss' 307–312
hormonal factors 50–51
hormone replacement
  therapy (HRT) 60
hyaluronic acid (HA)
  injections 219
5-hydroxytryptamine (5-HT)
  see serotonin
hyperglycaemia 132
hypertension *see* high
  blood pressure
hyponatremia 136, 139

ikigai *293*–295
immune system 46–47
  foods to boost 123–124
incidental activity 204–205
industry experts 271–273
inflammaging 124, 165
inflammation 164–166

foods to fight 124–125
  red wine 300
injection therapy 218–219
inner (holistic) health 40
insomnia 182–183
insulin 132–133
insulin resistance 132–133
intention-behaviour gap 80
iron, for women's health 59–60

jet lag 228–230
joint health 212–213
joint osteoarthritis 220
joint realignment
  surgery 219–220
joint replacement surgery 220

Krebs cycle 106

'laughter is the best
  medicine' 295–297
Lifeline 64
lipase 173
listener receptor deficit (LRD)
  condition 55, 199
long-term sleep deprivation
  177
love hormone *see* oxytocin
low blood pressure 35
low-density lipoprotein
  (LDL) 129
lung cancer 28–31
lymphocyte immune system 46

male deaths, in Australia 6

marriage 286–288

mastication 172–174

medical screening 84–86

Mediterranean
    diet 152, 153–156

Men's health
    ASOSS and 54–55
    avoiding health
        check-ups 52–53
    mental health
        issues for 62–64
    overview of 49–50
    prostate cancer 56–58
    vs. women 50–52

MensLine Australia 65

mental health 38–41
    for men and women 62–64
    telephone and online
        resources 64–65

Mental Health
    Commission of NSW 38

mentors 266–271

milk, for health 140–143

milk permeate 142

mindset
    attention to detail 260–261
    battles 276–278
    burnout 247–249
    children 252–254
    compassion 265–266
    don't be too hard on
        yourself 251–252

financial planning 274–276

goal setting 258–260

industry experts 271–273

keep learning 257–258

learn to adapt 278–280

mental state and improved
    health 239–240

mentor 266–271

moderation 283–284

never too early/late 280–282

practise gratefulness 254–255

procrastination 262–263

selfish 255–257

solitude 264

stress management 240–246

willpower 249–251

mitochondria 5, 105–108

moderation 283–284

monounsaturated fats 129

Moodgym 65

muscle tone 82

music 304–305

NAD *see* nicotinamide adenine
    dinucleotide (NAD)

National Health and Medical
    Research Council
    (NHMRC) 32

National Study of Mental
    Health and Wellbeing
    (2020-22) 62–63

'never judge a book by its
    cover' 315–317

nicotinamide adenine
  dinucleotide
  (NAD) 108–109
nightmares 188–189
nutraceuticals 218
nutrition
  alcohol consumption 150–151
  avoid processed foods 125–126
  avoid sugar 130–132
  body and brain, foods
    for 118–125
  chocolate 133–135
  coffee 143–146
  convenience food 114
  description of 113
  diets 151–152
  eat most/plenty/
    regularly/less 120
  fasting and timed
    eating 161–163
  fluid intake and
    hydration 137
  food labelling 171–172
  fuel intake 117–118
  good carbohydrates 126–127
  good fats *vs.* bad fats 128–129
  gut health 114–117
  healthy, sustainable
    weight 152–153
  inflammation 164–166
  mastication 172–174
  Mediterranean diet 153–156
  milk 140–143
  protein 127–128
  rainbow principle 157–158
  salt 135–136
  snacks 163
  supplements 166–171
  tea 148–150
  water 137–140

obsessive-compulsive
  personality
  disorder (OCD) 261
obstructive sleep apnoea *see*
  sleep apnoea
osteoarthritis 212–213
  arthroscopy 219
  crepitus 215
  deformity/malalignment 215
  functional capacity,
    reduction in 216
  guided resistance/strength
    training program 217
  injection therapy 218–219
  instability 215
  joint 220
  joint realignment
    surgery 219–220
  joint replacement surgery
    220
  load modification 217–218
  non-steroidal
    anti-inflammatories 217
  nutraceuticals 218
  pain 214

pain management 216–217

patient education 216

physical therapy 217

stiffness 214–215

stronger medications 217

swelling 214

weakness and fatigue
    215–216

weight loss 218

osteoporosis 60–61

Ovid 254

oxytocin 192–193

Paffenbarger, Ralph 111

parking habits 208–209

perimenopause 60

personal health 40

pets, for health 211–212

physical activity *see* exercise

placebo effect 170

polyphenols 299

polyunsaturated fats 129

portion distortion 117

postcodes 226

practise gratefulness 254–255

primary insomnia 183

processed foods,
    avoiding 125–126

procrastination 262–263

prostate cancer 56–58

prostate-specific
    antigen (PSA) 57

protein 127–128

Qlife 65

Queen's telegram 7–8

rainbow foods 157–158

ralking activity 279

rapid eye movement
    (REM) 179, 188

red wine 299–302

religion 273–274

reproductive health 59

resistance training 89–90

restless legs syndrome
    186–187

resveratrol 300

salt, for health 135–136

SANE Australia 65

saturated fats 129

seafood 309

seasonal affective disorder
    syndrome (SADS) 231

secondary insomnia 183

selfish 255–257

Selye, Hans 242

senescent cells 4

'sense of self' 40

serotonin 115, 193–194

'seven Ss', holiday with 307–312

seafood 309

sex 311–312

sipping 310

sleep 307–308

social reading 310–311

'seven Ss', holiday with
(*Continued*)
  sunshine 308
  sweating 309
sex 288–291, 311–312
sipping 310
skin protection 201–204
sleep 176–177, 307–308
  deficit/deprivation 181
  DOSE hormones 190–195
  dreaming 187–189
  hygiene 180–181
  insomnia 182–183
  monitoring 182
  optimal amount of 177–178
  phases of 178–179
  reasons for 177
  'restless legs' 186–187
  snoring 185–186
sleep apnoea 183–185
smallpox vaccination 234
smoking habits 198–201
snacks 163
snoring 185–186
social reading 310–311
solitude 264
sport hydration drinks 141
stairs 207–208
strength training
  joint pain 217
  on muscle tone, 82, 89–90
stress 240–241

  dealing with 245–246
  manifestations 243–244
  origin of 241–242
strokes 26–28
sugar 130–132
sunshine 230–232, 308
supplementary Ss 312–314
supplements 166–171
sweating 309
systolic blood pressure 33

tea, for health 148–150
telomeres 5
Therapeutic Goods
  Administration (TGA) 273
3-3-3 method 197
timed eating 161–163
trans fats 129
transient ischaemic
  attack (TIA) 27
type 1 diabetes 132
type 2 diabetes 132–133
tyrosine 191

vaccinations 233–235

water, for health 137–140
willpower 249–251
wine
  health benefits of
    drinking 297–298
  history of 298–299

red 299–302
vintages and
varietals 300–302
women's health
health issues for 58–61
mental health for 62–64
men *vs.* 50–52
overview of 49–50
physical appearance
pressures and 61–62
workout 314–315
World Economic Forum 7